The Conundrum
of Human Behavior
in the Social Environment

The Conundrum of Human Behavior in the Social Environment has been co-published simultaneously as *Journal of Human Behavior in the Social Environment*, Volume 10, Number 3 2004.

First published 2004 by
The Haworth Social Work Practice Press, 10 Alice Street, Binghamton, NY 13904-1580 USA

The Haworth Social Work Practice Press is an imprint of The Haworth Press, Inc., 10 Alice Street, Binghamton, NY 13904-1580 USA.

This edition published 2013 by Routledge

Routledge
Taylor & Francis Group
711 Third Avenue
New York, NY 10017

Routledge
Taylor & Francis Group
2 Park Square, Milton Park
Abingdon, Oxon OX14 4RN

Routledge is an imprint of the Taylor & Francis Group, an informa business

The Conundrum of Human Behavior in the Social Environment has been co-published simultaneously as *Journal of Human Behavior in the Social Environment*, Volume 10, Number 3 2004.

© 2004 by The Haworth Press, Inc. All rights reserved. No part of this work may be reproduced or utilized in any form or by any means, electronic or mechanical, including photocopying, microfilm and recording, or by any information storage and retrieval system, without permission in writing from the publisher.

The development, preparation, and publication of this work has been undertaken with great care. However, the publisher, employees, editors, and agents of The Haworth Press and all imprints of The Haworth Press, Inc., including The Haworth Medical Press® and The Pharmaceutical Products Press®, are not responsible for any errors contained herein or for consequences that may ensue from use of materials or information contained in this work. Opinions expressed by the author(s) are not necessarily those of The Haworth Press, Inc.

Cover design by Jennifer M. Gaska.

Library of Congress Cataloging-in-Publication Data

The conundrum of human behavior in the social environment/Marvin D. Feit, John S. Wodarski, editors.
    p. cm.
"Co-published simultanously as Journal of human behavior in the social environment, volume 10, number 3 2004."
Includes bibliographical references and index.
    ISBN-10: 0-7890-2884-0 (hard cover: alk. paper)
    ISBN-13: 978-0-7890-2884-6 (hard cover: alk. paper)
    ISBN-10: 0-7890-2885-9 (soft cover: alk. paper)
    ISBN-13: 978-0-7890-2885-3 (soft cover: alk. paper)
1. Social work education. 2. Social service–Psychological aspects 3. Human behavior–Study and teaching (Higher). 4. Social psychology–Study and teaching (Higher) I. Feit, Marvin, D. II. Wodarski, John S. III. Journal of human behavior in the social environment.
HV11.C71863 2005
302'.071'–dc22
    2005001199

The Conundrum of Human Behavior in the Social Environment

Marvin D. Feit, PhD
John S. Wodarski, PhD
Editors

The Conundrum of Human Behavior in the Social Environment has been co-published simultaneously as *Journal of Human Behavior in the Social Environment*, Volume 10, Number 3 2004.

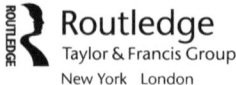

The Conundrum of Human Behavior in the Social Environment

CONTENTS

A Curriculum for Human Behavior in the Social Environment   1
    Tracy L. Zaparanick
    John S. Wodarski

Towards a Comprehensive Framework
   for Understanding the Social Environment:
   In Search of Theory for Practice   25
    Elizabeth A. Mulroy
    Michael J. Austin

Evaluating the Social Environment Component
   of Social Work Courses on Human Behavior
   and the Social Environment   61
    Sarah Taylor
    Michael J. Austin
    Elizabeth A. Mulroy

Social Work Textbooks on Human Behavior
   and the Social Environment: An Analysis
   of the Social Environment Component   85
    Sarah Taylor
    Elizabeth A. Mulroy
    Michael J. Austin

Reflecting on the Social Environment Dimensions
   of HB&SE: An HB&SE Faculty Member as Discussant   111
    Susan Stone

Index   119

ABOUT THE EDITORS

Marvin D. Feit, PhD, is Dean and Professor of the Norfolk State University Ethelyn R. Strong School of Social Work in Norfolk, VA. He is the author or co-author of several books and has written many articles and chapters in the areas of group work, substance abuse, health, and practice. Dr. Feit has made numerous presentations at national, state, and local conferences and has served as a consultant to profit and non-profit organizations, federal and state government agencies, and numerous community-based agencies. He is the founding Editor of the *Journal of Health & Social Policy* (The Haworth Press, Inc.) and of the *Journal of Human Behavior in the Social Environment* (The Haworth Press, Inc.).

John S. Wodarski, PhD, received his BS degree from Florida State University, the MSSW degree from the University of Tennessee, and the PhD degree from Washington University in Saint Louis. His main research interests include; child and adolescent health behavior, including research on violence, substance abuse, depression, sexuality, and employment. Dr. Wodarski is the author of 56 texts and over 500 journal publications. He received the Trailblazers Award from African American Authors in recognition of his work with minority populations. He has presented his research at over 275 professional meetings and conferences. Over the course of his career, Dr. Wodarski has been the recipient of 138 federal, state, institutional, and private foundation research awards. Dr. Wodarski currently serves as Co-Editor of the *Journal of Human Behavior in the Social Environment* and *Evidence-Based Social Work: Advances in Practice, Programming, Research, and Policy,* and is Editor-in-Chief of *Stress, Trauma, and Crisis: An International Journal.* He is Editor-in-Chief, The Haworth Press, Inc. *Social Work Series.* Dr. Wodarski's administrative experiences include serving as Principal Investigator of various grants; Director or Co-Director of three Research Centers; Department Chair; Director of two doctoral programs; and Associate Vice President for Graduate Studies and Research. Dr. Wodarski holds the title of Professor of Social Work at the University of Tennessee College of Social Work.

A Curriculum for Human Behavior in the Social Environment

Tracy L. Zaparanick
John S. Wodarski

SUMMARY. Consensus has not been reached regarding the content of human behavior in the social environment (HBSE) courses in schools of social work. Changes in the CSWE Education Policy and Accreditation Standards reflect, in part, the needs of the people social workers serve and the tools necessary to properly equip social workers in that pursuit. While considering the degree of dissension and change within the academic environment, theories of intervention should also provide the practitioner with an understanding of how detrimental behavior develops as well as how undesirable behaviors can be modified or eliminated. It also must provide a description of normal as well as dysfunctional behavior. It is crucial, therefore, that any theory of behavioral change identify the antecedent conditions through which the disordered behavior was acquired. It also must provide very specific behavioral prescriptions and procedures that the practitioner can use to eliminate the undesirable behaviors. An indispensable component of any educational program is the development of critical thinking skills. The HBSE curriculum is no different, and especially requires the use of this skill. In order for students to properly evalu-

---

Tracy L. Zaparanick, MSSW, LCSW, and John S. Wodarski, PhD, are affiliated with the University of Tennessee, Knoxville, College of Social Work.

[Haworth co-indexing entry note]: "A Curriculum for Human Behavior in the Social Environment." Zaparanick, Tracy L., and John S. Wodarski. Co-published simultaneously in *Journal of Human Behavior in the Social Environment* (The Haworth Social Work Practice Press, an imprint of The Haworth Press, Inc.) Vol. 10, No. 3, 2004, pp. 1-24; and: *The Conundrum of Human Behavior in the Social Environment* (ed: Marvin D. Feit and John S. Wodarski) The Haworth Social Work Practice Press, an imprint of The Haworth Press, Inc., 2004, pp. 1-24. Single or multiple copies of this article are available for a fee from The Haworth Document Delivery Service [1-800-HAWORTH, 9:00 a.m. - 5:00 p.m. (EST). E-mail address: docdelivery@haworthpress.com].

© 2004 by The Haworth Press, Inc. All rights reserved.
Digital Object Identifier: 10.1300/J137v10n03_01

ate the theories put before them while in the classroom or in practice, instruction must be given on how to evaluate and students given subsequent opportunities to apply these instructions. This article will focus on the micro and macro evidence-based curriculum, a new educational standard under the Council of Social Work Education, in the human behavior in the social environment module. *[Article copies available for a fee from The Haworth Document Delivery Service: 1-800-HAWORTH. E-mail address: <docdelivery@haworthpress.com> Website: <http://www.HaworthPress.com> © 2004 by The Haworth Press, Inc. All rights reserved.]*

KEYWORDS. Human behavior curriculum, materials, resources, innovations

Consensus has not been reached regarding the content of human behavior in the social environment courses in schools of social work (Farley, Smith, Boyle, & Ronnau, 2002; Gibbs, 1986). Courses become ineffective when students superficially review much of the same content in preceding degree programs and are especially problematic when students are provided few academic exercises which would enable them to witness the application of concepts to practice phenomenon. This article will focus on the evidence-based curriculum, a new educational standard under the Council of Social Work Education (CSWE, 2002), in the human behavior in the social environment (HBSE) module. Teaching methods and an exemplar syllabus will conclude this suggested curriculum for an evidence-based HBSE course.

Prior to 1915 the social work profession had already begun creating and training in empirical methodologies to explain human development in the social environment, while simultaneously recognizing the uniqueness of each person and their circumstances (Dolgoff & Feldstein, 2003). For instance, during The Milford Conference members assigned generic social casework as having several common themes which were to include the "established methods of study and treatment of human beings in need; and the adaptation of scientific knowledge and formulations of experience to the requirements of social casework" (Dolgoff & Feldstein, 2003, p. 311). Charity Organizations found strength in pledging empiricism to pauperism (Axinn & Levin, 1995). Despite the conceptual foundations of the social work profession the unfortunate gap between science and practice interventions continues to polarize the profession (Thyer, 1996; Wamback, Haynes, & White,

1999; Witkin, 1991). This opposition perpetually yields few methodological studies on the paradigms used in any social work practice compendium.

In 1952, the National Association of Schools of Social Administration merged with the American Association of Schools of Social Work to become the Council on Social Work Education (NASW, 1998). The CSWE is defined as:

> ... a national association that preserves and enhances the quality of social work education for practice that promotes the goals of individual and community well-being and social justice. CSWE pursues this mission through setting and maintaining policy and program standards, accrediting bachelor's and master's degree programs in social work, promoting research and faculty development, and advocating for social work education. (CSWE, 2003)

Changes in the CSWE Education Policy and Accreditation Standards reflect, in part, the needs of the people social workers serve and the tools necessary to properly equip social workers in that pursuit. For instance, in the CSWE 4th edition, additions were made to the HBSE curriculum standards to include: (1) the impact of social and economic forces on individuals and social systems; (2) examining how systems impact the well-being of the population being served; (3) integrate social work values and ethical issues regarding the bio-psycho-social theories; and (4) educate students how to critically evaluate theories and their applications to client situations (CSWE, 1994).

Comparing and contrasting the 4th edition to the most current 5th edition, the following items were added: (1) courses are to include empirically based theories; (2) include spiritual development theories across the life span; and (3) include the interplay between individuals and their environments (CSWE, 2002). Exclusions consisted of: (1) the impact of social and economic forces on individuals and social systems; (2) integrating values and ethical issues relating to social work practice; and (3) developing the skill of critically analyzing theories and their applications to client situations (CSWE, 1994). Of particular interest for this article is the directive to embrace empirical-based theories.

An indispensable component of any educational program is the development of critical thinking skills. The HBSE curriculum is no different, and especially requires the use of this skill. In order for students to properly evaluate the theories put before them while in the classroom or in practice, instruction must be given on how to evaluate and students given subsequent opportunities to apply these instructions. The intent of the instruction is to acquire and master such skills. Analogous to teaching critical thinking skills would be teaching the students how to fish, rather than just giving them the fish.

LITERATURE REVIEW FOR EVIDENCE-BASED HBSE CURRICULUM

The HBSE course is intended to provide students an applicable framework in order to describe, explain and ultimately predict human behavior, while taking into consideration the intricate and complex nature of each individual. The art of predicting human behavior has yet to be perfected; there is not one universal, all encompassing theory that can explain and subsequently forecast the actions of people. The best social science can do presently is offer various methods of conceptualizing the person-in-environment, some of which have been researched. There are a multitude of theories in existence; some have maintained through the test of time, while others have been replaced with more contemporary speculations. The cumulative literature to date lacks sufficient empirical depth for a HBSE course to be taught solely on the merits of evidence-based practice alone. The following section will identify what experimental literature exists for the micro and macro HBSE curriculum. An excellent resource for this course is *Human Behavior in the Social Environment–Integrating Theory and Evidence-Based Practice* by Wodarski and Dziegielewki (2002). This section will briefly summarize this compilation.

Individual Perspective to Human Growth and Development–Micro Issues

Biology and Genetics

Development of a course that focuses on the individual must consider a host of variables simultaneously to help determine what drives thoughts, feelings and actions of each individual. The connection between the mind and body continues to build momentum as the advances in medical technology and science uncover the biology of the individual, especially as it wonders about the physiological impact of stress and emotions (Carter, 1999; Lazarus, 1999; McEwen, 2002; Pert, 1999). Lawrence and Zittel-Palamara (2002) explore the influence of biology and genetics as it related to human growth and development. What follows is a list of theories and subsequent citations they use to illustrate the respective theory. These theories have tested the theoretical underpinnings to examine the extent of their applicability.

- Nature vs. Nurture
  - Influence of environmental factors in the development of psychopathology (Bellack & Mueser, 1993; Kendler & Deihl, 1993; Tsuang, 2000)
  - Maternal environment and attitude identified as risk factors regarding fetal outcomes (Gennaro, Brooten, Roncoli, & Kumar, 1993; Mednick et al., 1998)
  - Mood disorders (Kaplan, Saddock, & Grebb, 1994)
  - Alcoholism (Farren & O'Malley, 1999)
  - Suicide (Brent, 1995; Brent et al., 1993; Gottesman, 1991)
- General Adaptation Syndrome (Selye, 1956)
  - Correlation between stress and headaches (DeBenedittis & Loren-zetti, 1992)
  - Physical maladies are lifestyle-related (Ell & Northern, 1990)
  - Psychological stress may induce migraines (Henryk-Gritt & Rees, 1973)
  - Associations between work-related stress and the well-being of the employee (Bosma, Peter, Siegrist, & Marmot, 1998; Sorensen, Lewis, & Bishop, 1996)
  - Relationship between stress and asthmatic symptoms (Janson-Bjerklie, Ferkeitch, & Brenner, 1993)
  - The rise of stress associated conditions, both physical & mental (Greenberg, Stiglin, Finkelstein, & Berndt, 1993)
- Aggression (Rothenburg, 1975)
  - Hereditary factors and aggression in animals (Goldstein, 1974)
  - Criminality and twins (Dilalla & Gottesman, 1991)
  - Testosterone and aggression (Booth & Osgood, 1993, Coccaro, Kavoussi, & McNamee, 2000)
- Personality types (Bulbulian & Bitters, 1996; Monforton, Helmes, & Deathe, 1993)
  - Type A personality and coronary artery disease (Carmelli, Rosenman, Chesney, Gabsitz, Lee, & Borhani, 1988; Espnes & Opdahl, 1999)

Cognitive Theory

In the continuing effort to interpret and predict human behavior, cognitive theorists expand on behaviorism. Rather than limiting the individual to simply responding to a stimulus, an additional element of cognition has been identified (Bolles, 1974; McCarthy & Rude, 2000). It is believed that cognition encompasses not only the interpretation of a particular event, but can also evoke a response simply through imagination or anticipation of a feared event (Folkman, Schaefer, & Lazarus, 1979). Dulmus (2002) provides a comprehensive resource for empirical-based cognitive and cognitive-behavioral theories. Below is a listing of some of her supporting studies:

- Cognitive Theory (Beck, Rush, Shaw, & Emery, 1979; Goodwin & Guze, 1989)
  - Cognitive therapy and psychiatric disorders (Breitholtz, Johansson, & Ott, 1999; Salkovskis, 1999)
- Cognitive-Behavioral Theory (Kendall, 1991)
  - Cognitive-behavioral therapy (Gortner, Gollan, Dobson, & Jacobson, 1998; Kendall & Panichelli-Mindel, 1995; Murphy, Carney, Knesevich, & Whitworth, 1995)
  - Assessment, diagnosis, and treatment (Dulmus & Wodarski, 1998; Finch, Nelson, & Ott, 1993)

Life Span Perspective

Life span development theorists contend that as individuals navigate throughout life, development remains constant. Social workers realizing the impact of various life stages understand that this calls for a decision from various interventions. Consequently, the intervention is embedded in the understanding of these life stages. In Dwyer and Hunt-Jackson (2002), each life stage is covered in depth and potential scenarios social workers may find themselves in. Within their chapter, they offer suggested readings for each stage. The list below targets only a few of those articles.

- Life Span Theory–Piaget, Bowlby, and Erickson (Belsky, Lerner, & Spanier, 1984)
  - Prenatal Development (Hayes & Batshaw, 1993)
  - Infants and Toddlers (Quinn, 1998)
  - Early Childhood (Feldman, Caplinger, & Wodarski, 1983)

- Later Childhood (Eron, Huesmann, Dubow, Romanoff, & Yarmel, 1987)
- Adolescence (Hoffman, Paris, & Hall, 1994)
- Early Adulthood (Lefrancois, 1993)
- Middle Adulthood (Goleman, 1990)
- Later Adulthood (Chima, 2002; Cui & Vaillant, 1996; Sherr, 2002)

Labeling Theory

Interventions should be based on the clearly defined need or problem. The social sciences provide social workers numerous instruments so to arrive at the identified problem more accurately and efficiently. The strategy to alleviate the need can then be prepared. However, the exactness of the identified problem area is contingent upon the accuracy of the instrument and subsequent interpretation and perception of the results. Perception is a primary driver of the hypothesis-testing theory (Bruner, 1951, 1957; Postman, 1951). Labeling a client can have several serious, albeit adverse implications for the labeled. Sullivan (2002) cites several instances of these implications:

- Labeling Theory (Lemert, 1951, 1967)
  - Professional training contributions and bias (Quicke & Winter, 1994)
  - Inaccurate labeling (Gingerich, Feldman, & Wodarski, 1976a, 1976b)
  - Deviant labeling (Schmid & Jones, 1991; Stager, Chassin, & Young, 1983)
  - Labeling and outcomes (Link, 1987; Link, Cullen, Sturening, Shrout, & Dohrenwend, 1989)
  - Expectancy biases (Ysseldyke & Algozzine, 1981)
  - Stigmatizing labels (Haring & Lovetti, 1992)

Group Perspective to Human Growth and Development

Learning Theories

Integrating how humans theoretically respond to pleasure and pain increases the probability of inducing behavioral changes (Iverson, 1992). The operant respondent model predicts human behavior by calculating the likelihood of certain behaviors being duplicated or extinguished based on events just prior to behavior (antecedent events) and the potential consequences of the displayed behavior (Moote, Skiba, & Hall, 2002). Classical conditioning draws its strength from creating a strong association between an event/object and a negative/positive response. The observational paradigm stems from the social learning school. This observational modeling framework claims learning can be completed vicariously. Referencing the work by Moote et al. (2002), these extracted citations may be used in the classroom.

- Operant Theory (Skinner, 1953, 1969)
  - Reinforcing behaviors with couples (Bagarozzi & Wodarski, 1978; Wodarski, 1997)
  - Influence of persuasive communication (Strathman, Gleicher, Boninger, & Edwards, 1994)
  - Autistic children and increases in social behaviors (Hamblin, Buckholdt, Ferritor, Kozloff, & Blackwell, 1971)
  - Reducing unacceptable behaviors in children (Lalli, Casey, & Kates, 1995)
- Respondent Theory (Pavlov, 1927)
  - Classical conditioning (Watson & Rayner, 1920)
  - Phobias and anxiety (King, 1993; Schneider & Nevid, 1993)
- Modeling Theory (Bandura, Adams, & Beyer, 1977)
  - Vicarious learning (Kazdin, 1989; Ladoucer, 1983)

Social Exchange

The social exchange theory provides insights by acknowledging and taking into account the exchange between people and their social context, whether it is another individual or an organization. Based on the integration of behavioral theories, the social exchange theory is defined by the schedules of reinforcement. These include continuous, fixed-interval, fixed ration, variable-ratio, and variable-interval (Rapp-Pagilicci, 2002). The following briefly summarizes the work by Rapp-Pagilicci (2002).

- Schedules of reinforcement (Long, Hammack, May, & Campbell, 1958; Salzinger, 1969)
  - Range of applicability (Lawler & Thye, 1999)
  - Continuous reinforcement (Elkind, 1971)
  - Therapeutic relationships (Molm, Quist, & Wisely, 1994)
  - Concealment of negative qualities (Early, 1992)

- Social worker burnout (Dressel, Waters, Sweat, & Clayton, 1990)

Group Level Variables

Reviewing Yalom's (1995) pivotal work in the theory and practice of group therapy illustrates the utility it has in social work practice. Motivations to facilitate group interventions range from the cost-effectiveness of serving several individuals at once to what Bowman and Delucia (1993) describe as creating a small social environment so members can experiment with newly acquired social skills. Despite the catalyst for group work, it has transformed the face of mental health services. Smith, Leo, and Maccio (2002) introduce multiple research efforts to examine the applicability and effectiveness of group theory. What follows was taken from their work.

- Group Theory (Levine, 1991; Wodarski & Feit, 1994; Yalom, 1995)
  - Homogeneity within a group (Williams, 1994)
  - Out-group homogeneity variable (Smith, Tindale, & Dugoni, 1996)
  - In-group homogeneity (Lee & Ottati, 1995)
  - Diversity within work groups (Bantz, 1993)
  - Preferences of ethnic-specific groups (Chu & Sue, 1984; Davis & Proctor, 1989)
  - Schizophrenia and higher level functioning groups (Beeber, 1991)
  - Meta-analysis on homogeneity-heterogeneity benefits (Bowers, Pharmer, & Salas, 2000)
  - Group cohesion (Braaten, 1989; Wright & Duncan, 1986)
  - Leadership (Albright & Forziati, 1995; Stinchfield & Burlingame, 1991)

Macro-Level Variables

Influences on human behavior that are not addressed by individual or group interventions are thought to be "macro" in nature. Accordingly, macro-level social work addresses the organizational and communal arenas as it relates to the policies and procedures therein. Heightening students' awareness of social, political, historical, economic, and environmental influences bring clarity to the person-in-environment standard. Dziegieleski and Wodarski (2002) inform the reader of the impact macro-level variables have on the social work profession. Listed below are examples taken from their work.

- Macro-related issues (Colby & Dziegielewski, 2001; Kirst-Ashman & Hull, 1997; Zastrow, 1999)
  - Minority groups and vulnerable populations (Cohen & Wagner, 1992; DuBois & Miley, 1999; Mulroy & Lane, 1992; See, 1998)
  - Change agents and social change strategies (Miceli, 1984)
  - Discriminatory practices (Dozier & Miceli, 1985; Herzog, 1971; Smith, 1973)
  - Impact of economic declines (Hamburg, 1994; Weinert, 1982)

IMPLICATIONS FOR HBSE CURRICULUM

The aforementioned concepts can be covered in a two-semester course. The first semester course may focus on dyadic interaction and the second on small group interaction, however, both courses should include impact of organizations and communities within the social, political, historical, economic, and environmental contexts. Students should be able to make decisions as to whether or not the concepts are adequate for social work practice through employing the scientific and practice criteria. Classroom activities are presented in Appendix 1. These experiences provide students the opportunity to exchange ideas regarding the application and evaluation of concepts. The application of a particular concept to bring about change in the client, i.e., individual, group, and/or organization is demonstrated.

Two critical skills students and practitioners must possess for successful practice endeavors which are based on a rational, empirical basis are the ability to evaluate research studies and the ability to translate research into practice generalizations (Fischer, 1978a, 1978b). Given the extent of theoretical perspectives, strengthening critical thinking skills is a necessary component to any social work curriculum.

A critical consideration when selecting a theory of human behavior and personality development is whether or not the speculative concept has had any prior empirical screening (Fischer, 1971; Wodarski & Feldman, 1973). This criterion cannot be compromised by a profession with an historical tradition of dedication to the promotion of human welfare and commitment to a specific method of inquiry. Theories used in practice should have their day in empirical court. Not only must the theory be capable of describing and explaining the phenomena under consideration, but it must also have the power to predict those phenomena accurately and reliably so that they can be controlled and manipulated to produce desired behavioral changes. A requisite for theories used in practice should successfully withstand numerous empirical tests of its tenets and hypotheses like its counterparts that claim the power to induce change. In other words, concepts used in practice should undergo the same evaluative methods by which all scientific theories are judged.

Any theory of intervention should provide the practitioner with an understanding of how detrimental behavior develops as well as how undesirable behaviors can be modified or eliminated. It also must provide a description of normal as well as dysfunctional behavior. It is crucial, therefore, that any theory of behavioral change identify the antecedent conditions through which the disordered behavior was acquired. It also must provide very specific behavioral prescriptions and procedures that the practitioner can use to eliminate the undesirable behaviors.

Unfortunately, the field of social work has not traditionally adhered to such criteria for the selection of its knowledge base. As a result, practice theories and intervention techniques with unknown empirical effectiveness have been passed down from one generation of clinical practitioners to the next. The practice of consciously excluding theories of human behavior and clinical practice whose efficacy have substantial empirical support from the curricula of schools of social work in favor of theories that have little or no scientific backing cannot help the profession to attain its mission.

Basic human behavior courses should be offered at the undergraduate level. These should include an introduction to human behavior focusing on the dyad and a course centering on the use of groups in human service practice and the effect of the worker on various organizational groupings. Additionally, all students should have an introductory course in cultural diversity to enable the understanding of the various minority groups that a social work practitioner encounters. These three courses provide some basic prerequisites for practice. The contribution of doctoral education to the HBSE coursework would be to assist students in the instruction of testing these human behavior concepts.

The investigation of effective teaching methods within the HBSE curriculum has to date three empirical studies (Johnson & Rhodes, 2001; Spero, 1982; Sutton, 1981). The latter two references utilized the pre-post test design to measure the retention of HBSE course content, using an interactive and/or didactic instruction style. Findings indicate that both serve the students equally well. Johnson and Rhodes (2001) solicited feedback from MSW students regarding the applicability of course content. Improvements were noted in the textbook coverage in social justice and strengths perspectives for at-risk populations. These studies are just the beginning of how and what needs to be implemented in the HBSE curriculum. Reyes (2002) has outlined course objectives and simulations exercises within an evidence-based HBSE course. With the explosion of Internet-access computers, teaching trends are changing on campuses. Many are considering how this technology may replace traditional attendance driven courses with distance learning options in social work (Faux & Black-Hughes, 2000; Johnson & Huff, 2000; Menon & Coe, 2000; Petracchi, 2000; Schoech, 2000; Stocks & Freddolino, 2000). Effects of media technology on social work students are also at a primitive but thriving stage (Cauble & Thurston, 2000; Huff, 2000; Vinton & Harrington, 1994).

CONCLUSION

Adhering to the CSWE standards are critical to any accredited program. This article hopes to be a resource of what theories will meet the evidence-based theory requirement in the most recent educational policy and accreditation standards. Exposure to critical thinking skills should be a perquisite to the HBSE coursework and strengthen throughout this course-sequence curriculum. Proliferation in interest and movement toward empirical-based practice holds a promise of multiple options for the educator, student and practitioner.

REFERENCES

Albright, L., & Forziati, C. (1995). Cross-sectional consistency and perceptual accuracy in leadership. *Personality and Social Psychology Bulletin*, 21(12), 1269-1276.
Axinn, J., & Levin, H. (1995). *Social Welfare: A History of the American Response to Need*. New York: Longman.
Bagarozzi, D. A., & Wodarski, J. S. (1978). Behavioral treatment of marital discord. *Clinical Social Work Journal*, 6(2), 135-154.
Bandura, A., Adams, N. E., & Beyer, J. (1977). Cognitive processes mediating behavioral change. *Journal of Personality & Social Psychology*, 3(5), 125-139.
Bantz, C. R. (1993). Cultural diversity and group cross-cultural team research. *Journal of Applied Communication Research*, 21(1), 1-20.

Beck, A. T., Rush, A. J., Shaw, B. F., & Emery, G. (1979). *Cognitive therapy of depression*. New York: Guilford Press.
Beeber, A. R. (1991). Psychotherapy with schizophrenics in Team Groups: A systems model. *American Journal of Psychotherapy*, 45(1), 78-86.
Bellack, A. S., & Mueser, K. T. (1993). Psychosocial treatment for schizophrenia. In D. Shore (Ed.), *Schizophrenia*. Washington, DC: U.S. Government Printing Office.
Belsky, J., Lerner, R., & Spanier, G. (1984). *The child in the family*. Redding, MA: Addison-Welsey.
Bolles, R. C. (1974). Cognition and motivation: Some historical trends. In B. Weiner (Ed.), *Cognitive views of human motivation*. New York: Academic.
Booth, A., & Osgood, D. W. (1993). The influence of testosterone on deviance in adulthood: Assessing and explaining the relationship. *Criminology*, 31, 91-117.
Bosma, H., Peter, R., Siegrist, L., & Marmot, M. (1998). Two alternative job stress models and the risk of coronary heart disease. *American Journal of Public Health*, 88(1), 68-74.
Bowers, C. A., Pharmer, J. A., & Salas, E. (2000). When member homogeneity is needed in work teams: A meta-analysis. *Small Group Research*, 31(3), 305-327.
Bowman, V. E., & Delucia, J. L. (1993). Preparation for group therapy: The effects of preparer and modality on group process and individual functioning. *Journal for Specialists in Group Work*, 18(2), 67-79.
Braaten, L. J. (1989). Predicting positive goal attainment and symptom reduction from early group climate dimensions. *International Journal of Group Psychotherapy*, 39(3 Special Issue), 377-387.
Breitholtz, E., Johansson, B., & Ost, L. (1999). Cognitions in generalized anxiety disorder and panic disorder patients: A prospective approach. *Behaviour Research and Therapy*, 37(6), 533-544.
Brent, D. A. (1995). Risk factors for adolescent suicide and suicidal behavior: Mental and substance abuse disorders, family environmental factors, and life stress. *Suicide and Life-Threatening Behavior*, 25, Supplement, 52-63.
Brent, D. A., Perper, J. A., Moritz, G., Baugher, M., Roth, C., Balach, L., & Schweers, J. (1993). Stressful life events, psychopathology, and adolescent suicide: A case control study. *Suicide and Life-Threatening Behavior*, 23(3), Fall, 179-187.
Bruner, J. G. (1951). Personality dynamics and the process of perceiving. In R. Blake, & G. Ramsey (Eds.), *Perceptions: An approach to personality*. New York: Ronald Press.
Bruner, J.G. (1957). On perceptual readiness. *Psychological Review*, 64, 123-152.
Bulbulian, R., & Bitters, D. (1996). Blood pressure response to acute exercise in Type A and B females and males. *Physiology & Behavior*, 60(4), 1177-1182.
Carmelli, D., Rosenman, R., Chesney, M., Fabsitz, R., Lee, M., & Borhani, N. (1988). Genetic heritability and shared environmental influences of Type A measures in the NHLBI twin study. *American Journal of Epidemiology*, 127(6), 1041-1052.
Carter, R. (1999). *Mapping the Mind*. Berkeley, CA: University of California Press.
Cauble, A. E., & Thurston, L. P. (2000). Effects of Interactive Multimedia Training on Knowledge, Attitudes, and Self-Efficacy of Social Work Students. *Research on Social Work Practice*, 10(4), 428-437.

Chima, F. O. (2002). Elderly Suicidality: Human Behavior and Social Environment Perspective. *Journal of Human Behavior in the Social Environment*, 6(4), 21-46.

Chu, J., & Sue, S. (1984). Asian/Pacific-American and group practice. *Social Work with Groups*, 7(3), 23-36.

Coccaro, E. F., Kavoussi, R. J., & McNamee, B. (2000). Central neurotransmitter function in criminal aggression. In D. H. Fishbein (Ed.), *The science, treatment, and prevention of antisocial behaviors: Application to the criminal justice system*. Kingston, NJ: Civic Research Institute.

Cohen, M. B., & Wagner, D. (1992). Acting on their own behalf: Affiliation and political mobilization among homeless people. *Journal of Sociology & Social Welfare*, 19(4), 21-39.

Colby, I., & Dziegielewski, S. F. (2001). *Introduction to social work: The people's profession*. Chicago: Lyceum.

Council on Social Work Education–Commission on Accreditation. (1994). *Handbook of Accreditation Standards and Procedures* (4th Edition). Alexandria, VA: Author

Council on Social Work Education. (November, 2002). *Education Policy and Accreditation Standards*. Retrieved February 3, 2003, from *http://www.cswe.org/* (follow path–accreditation/New EPAS/pdf.doc).

Council on Social Work Education. (November, 2003). *What is CSWE?* Retrieved February 3, 2003, from *http://www.cswe.org/* (follow path–about CSWE/FAQ).

Cui, X., & Vaillant, G. E. (1996). Antecedents and consequences of negative life events in adulthood: A longitudinal study. *American Journal of Psychiatry*, 153(1), 21-26.

Davis, L., & Proctor, E. (1989). *Race, gender, and class: Guidelines for practice with individuals, families, and groups*. Englewood Cliffs, NJ: Prentice-Hall.

DeBenedittis, G., & Lorenzetti, A. (1992). Minor stressful life events (daily hassles) in chronic primary headache: Relationship with MMPI personality patterns. *Headache*, 32(7), 330-334.

Dilalla, L. F., & Gottesman, I. I. (1991). Biological and genetic contributors to violence–Wisdom's untold tale. *Psychological Bulletin*, 109(1), 125-129.

Dolgoff, R., & Feldstein, D. (2003). *Understanding Social Welfare*. Boston, MA: Allyn and Bacon.

Dozier, J. B., & Miceli, J. P. (1985). Potential predictors of whistle blowing: A prosocial behavior perspective. *Academy of Management Review*, 10(4), 823-836.

Dressel, P., Waters, M., Sweat, M., & Clayton, O. (1990). Exchange rules in the mediation of social welfare work. *Journal of Sociology & Social Welfare*, 17(4), 75-97.

DuBois, B., & Miley, K. K. (1999). *Social work: An empowering profession*. Needham Heights, MA: Allyn and Bacon.

Dulmus, C. N. (2002). Cognitive Variables as Factors in Human Growth and Development. In J. S. Wodarski, & S. F. Dziegielewki (Eds.), *Human Behavior in the Social Environment–Integrating Theory and Evidence-Based Practice* (pp. 64-83). New York: Springer Publishing.

Dulmus, C. N., & Wodarski, J. S. (1998). Major depressive disorder and dysthymic disorder. In B. Thyer, & J. S. Wodarski (Eds.), *Handbook of empirical social work practice* (Vol. 1), 273-285.

Dwyer, D., & Hunt-Jackson, J. (2002). The Life Span Perspective. In J. S. Wodarski & S. F. Dziegielewki (Eds.), *Human Behavior in the Social Environment–Integrating Theory and Evidence-Based Practice* (pp. 84-109). New York: Springer Publishing.

Dziegielewski, S. F., & Wodarski, J. S. (2002). Macro-Level Variables as Factors in Human Growth and Development. In J. S. Wodarski, & S. F. Dziegielewki (Eds.), *Human Behavior in the Social Environment–Integrating Theory and Evidence-Based Practice* (pp. 249-269). New York: Springer Publishing.

Early, B. (1992). An ecological-exchange model of social work consultation within the work group of the school. *Social Work in Education*, 14(4), 207-214.

Elkind, D. (Ed.). (1971). *Learning: An introduction*. Genview, IL: Scott and Foresman.

Ell, K., & Northern, H. (1990). *Families and heath care: Psychosocial practice*. New York: Aldine De Gruyer.

Eron, L., Huesmann, L., Dubow, E., Romanoff, R., & Yarmel, P. (1987). Aggression and its correlates over 22 years. In D. Crowell, I. Evans, & C. O'Donnell (Eds.), *Childhood aggression and violence*. New York: Plenum.

Espnes, G. A., & Opdahl, A. (1999). Association among behavior personality, and traditional risk factors for coronary heart disease: A study at a primary health center in mid-Norway. *Psychological Reports*, 85(2), 505-517.

Farley, O. W., Smith, L. L., Boyle, S. W., & Ronnau, J. (2002). A Review of Foundation MSW Human Behavior Courses. *Journal of Human Behavior in the Social Environment*, 6(2), 1-12.

Farren, C. K., & O'Malley, S. S. (1999). Occurrence and management of depression in the context of Naltrexone treatment of alcoholism. *American Journal of Psychiatry*, 156(8), 1258-1262.

Faux, T. L., & Black-Hughes, C. (2000). A Comparison of Using the Internet Versus Lectures to Teach Social Work History. *Research on Social Work Practice*, 10(4), 454-466.

Feldman, R., Caplinger, T., & Wodarski, J. (1983). *The St. Louis conundrum: The effective treatment of antisocial youths*. Englewood Cliffs, NJ: Prentice-Hall.

Finch, A. J., Nelson, W. M., & Ott, E. S. (1993). *Cognitive-behavioral procedures with children and adolescents*. Boston: Allyn and Bacon.

Fischer, J. (1971). A framework for the analysis and comparison of clinical theories of induced change. *Social Service Review*, 45, 110-130.

Fischer, J. (1978a). Does anything work? *Journal of Social Service Research*, 1(3), 215-243.

Fischer, J. (1978b). *Effective casework practice: An eclectic approach*. New York: McGraw-Hill.

Folkman, S., Schaefer, C., & Lazarus, R. (1979). Cognitive processes as mediators of stress and coping. In V. Hamilton, & D. Warburton (Eds.), *Human stress and cognition*. New York: Wiley.

Gennaro, S., Brooten, D., Roncoli, M., & Kumar, S. (1993). Stress and health outcomes among mothers of low-birthweight infants. *Western Journal of Nursing Research*, 15(1), 97-113.

Gibbs, P. (1986). HBSE in the Undergraduate Curriculum: A Survey. *Journal of Social Work Education*, 2, 46-52.

Gingerich, W., Feldman, R. A., & Wodarski, J.S. (1976a). Accurate and inaccurate attributions of anti-social behavior. A labeling perspective. *Sociological and Social Research*, 61, 204-222.

Gingerich, W., Feldman, R. A., & Wodarski, J.S. (1976b). Accuracy in assessment: Does training help? *Social Work*, 2(10), 40-48.

Goldstein, M. (1974). Brain research and violent behavior. *Archives of Neurology*, 30, 8-31.

Goleman, D. (1990, February 6). In midlife, not just crisis but care and comfort too. *New York Times*, pp. B5, B9.

Goodwin, D. W., & Guze, S. B. (1989). *Psychiatric diagnosis*. New York: Oxford University Press.

Gortner, E. T., Gollan, J. K., Dobson, K. S., & Jacobson, N. S. (1998). Cognitive-behavioral treatment for depression: Relapse prevention. *Journal of Consulting & Clinical Psychology*, 66(2), 377-384.

Gottesman, I. I. (1991). *Schizophrenia Genesis: The origins of madness*. New York: Freeman.

Greenburg, R. E., Stiglin, L. E., Finkelstein, S. N., & Berndt, E. R. (1993). The economic burden of depression in 1990. *Journal of Clinical Psychiatry*, 54(11), 405-418.

Hamblin, R. L., Buckholdt, D. R., Ferritor, D., Kozloff, M. A., & Blackwell, L. J. (1971). *The humanization process: A social behavioral analysis of children's problems*. New York: Wiley.

Hamburg, D. A. (1994). *Today's children: Creating a future for a generation in crisis*. New York: Times Books.

Haring, K. A., & Lovett, D. L. (1992). Labeling preschoolers as learning disabled: A cautionary position. *Topics in Early Childhood Special Education*, 12(2), 151-173.

Hayes, A., & Batshaw, M. L. (1993). Down Syndrome. *Pediatric Clinics of North America*, 40(3), 523-539.

Henryk-Gritt, S., & Rees, W. L. (1973). Psychological aspects of migraine. *Journal of Psychosomatic Research*, 17, 140-153.

Herzog, E. (1971). Who should be studies? *American Journal of Orthopsychiatry*, 16(1), 4-12.

Hoffman, L., Paris, S., & Hall, E. (1994). *Developmental psychology today*. New York: McGraw-Hill.

Huff, M. T. (2000). A Comparison Study of Live Instruction Versus Interactive Television for Teaching MSW Students Critical Thinking Skills. *Research on Social Work Practice*, 10(4), 400-416.

Iverson, I. H. (1992). Skinner's early research: From reflexology to operant conditioning. *American Psychologist*, 47(11), 1318-1328.

Janson-Bjerklie, S., Ferkeitch, S., & Benner, P. (1993). Predicting the outcomes of living with asthma. *Research in Nursing and Health*. 16(4), 241-250.

Johnson, M. M., & Huff, M. T. (2000). Student's Use of Computer-Mediated Communication in a Distance Education Course. *Research on Social Work Practice*, 10(4), 519-532.

Johnson, M. M., & Rhodes, R. (2001). "Give Me Strengths!" Evaluating the Effectiveness of a Graduate Level HBSE Course. *Journal of Human Behavior in the Social Environment*, 4(1), 1-18.

Kaplan, H. I., Saddock, B. J., & Grebb, J. A. (1994). *Synopsis of psychiatry: Behavioral sciences clinical psychiatry* (pp. 516-563). Baltimore: Williams & Wilkins.

Kazdin, A. E. (1989). *Behavior modification in applied settings* (4th ed.). Pacific Grove, CA: Brooks/Cole.

Kendall, P. C. (1991). *Child and adolescent therapy: Cognitive-behavior procedures*. New York: Guilford Press.

Kendall, P.C., & Panichelli-Mindel, S. M. (1995). Cognitive-behavioral treatments. *Journal of Abnormal Child Psychology*, 23(1), 107-123.

Kendler, K. S., & Diehl, S. R. (1993). The genetics of schizophrenia: A current, genetic epidemiological perspective. *Schizophrenia Bulletin*, 19(2), 261-286.

King, N. I. (1993). Simple and social phobias. *Advances in Clinical Child Psychology*, 15, 305-341.

Kirst-Ashman, K. K., & Hull, G. H., Jr. (1997). *Understanding generalist practice*. Chicago: Nelson-Hall.

Ladoucer, R. (1983). Participant modeling with or without cognitive treatment for phobias. *Journal of Consulting & Clinical Psychology*, 51, 930-932.

Lalli, J. S., Casey, S., & Kates, K. (1995). Reducing escape behavior and increasing task completion with functional communication training, extinction, and response chaining. *Journal of Applied Behavioral Analysis*, 28, 261-268.

Lawler, E., & Thye, S. (1999). Bringing emotion into social exchange theory. *Annual Review of Sociology*, 25, 217-244.

Lawrence, S. A., & Zittel-Palamara, K. (2002). The Interplay Between Biology, Genetics, and Human Behavior. In J. S. Wodarski, & S. F. Dziegielewki (Eds.), *Human Behavior in the Social Environment–Integrating Theory and Evidence-Based Practice* (pp. 39-63). New York: Springer Publishing.

Lazarus, R. (1999). *Stress and Emotion*. New York: Springer Publishing.

Lee, Y. T., & Ottati, V. (1995). Perceived in-group homogeneity as a function of group memberships alliance and stereotype threat. *Personality and Social Psychology Bulletin*, 21(6), 610-619.

Lefrancois, G. (1993). *The lifespan*. Belmont, CA: Wadsworth.

Lemert, E. (1951). *Social pathology: A systemic approach to the theory of sociopathic behavior*. New York: McGraw-Hill.

Lemert, E. M. (1967). *Human deviance, social problems, and social control*. Englewood Cliffs, NJ: Prentice-Hall.

Levine, B. (1991). *Group psychotherapy: Practice and development*. Prospect, IL: Waveland.

Link, B. (1987). Understanding labeling effects in the area of mental disorders: An assessment of the effects of expectations of rejection. *American Sociological Review*, 52, 96-112.

Link, B., Cullen, F., Struening, E., Shrout, P., & Dohrenwend, B. (1989). A modified labeling theory approach to mental disorders: An empirical assessment. *American Sociological Review*, 54, 400-423.

Long, E., Hammack, J., May, F., & Campbell, B. (1958). Intermittent reinforcement of operant behavior in children. *Journal of Experimental Analysis of Behavior*, 1(4), 315-339.

McCarthy, C., & Rude, S. (2000). Cognitively based counseling: Current state and future directions. *TCA Journal*, 28(1), 32-40.

McEwen, B. (with Lasley, E.N.). (2002). *The End of Stress as We Know It*. Washington, DC: Joseph Henry Press.

Mednick, S. A., Watson, J. B., Huttunen, M., Cannon, T. D., Katila, H., Machon, R., Mednic, B., Hollister, M., Parnas, J., Schulsinger, F., Sajaniemi, N., Voldsgaard, P., Pyhala, R., Gutkind, D., & Wang, X. (1998). A two-hit working model of the etiology of schizophrenia. In M.F. Lenzenweger, & R. H. Dworkin (Eds.), *Origins and development of schizophrenia: Advances in experimental psychopathology* (pp. 27-66). Washington, DC: American Psychological Association.

Menon, G. M., & Coe, J. A. (2000). Technology and Social Work Education: Recent Empirical Studies. *Research on Social Work Practice*, 10(4), 397-399.

Miceli, M. P. (1984). The relationships among beliefs, organizational position, and whistle blowing status: A discriminant analysis. *Academy of Management Journal*, 27(4), 687-705.

Molm, L., Quist, T., & Wisely, P. (1994). Imbalanced structures, unfair strategies: Power and justice in social exchange. *American Sociological Review*, 59, 98-121.

Monforton, M., Helmes, E., & Deathe, A. B. (1993). Type A personality and marital intimacy in amputees. *British Journal of Medical Psychology*, 66(10), 275-280.

Moote, G., Jr., Skiba, D., & Hall, J. (2002). Learning Theories: Their Application to Understanding Human Behavior. In J. S. Wodarski, & S. F. Dziegielewki (Eds.), *Human Behavior in the Social Environment–Integrating Theory and Evidence-Based Practice* (pp. 157-198). New York: Springer Publishing.

Mulroy, E. A., & Lane, T. S. (1992). Housing affordability, stress and single mothers: Pathway to homelessness. *Journal of Sociology & Social Welfare*, 19(3), 51-63.

Murphy, G. E., Carney, R. M., Knesevich, M. A., & Whitworth, P. (1995). Cognitive behavioral therapy, relaxation training, and tricyclic antidepressant medication in the treatment of depression. *Psychological Reports*, 77(2), 403-420.

National Association of Social Workers. (1998). *Milestones in the Development of Social Work and Social Welfare 1950s-Present*. Retrieved March 2, 2003, from *http://www.socialworkers.org/profession/centennial/milestones_4.htm*

Pavlov, I. P. (1927). *Conditioned Reflexes*. London, England: Clarendon Press.

Pert, C. B. (1999). *Molecules of Emotion*. New York: Touchstone.

Petracchi, H. E. (2000). Distance Education: What Do Our Students Tell Us? *Research on Social Work Practice*, 10(4), 362-376.

Postman, L. (1951). Toward a general theory of cognition. In J. Rohrer, & M. Sherif (Eds.), *Social psychology at the crossroads*. New York: Harper and Row.

Quicke, J., & Winter, C. (1994). A labeling and learning: An interaction perspective. *Support for Learning*, 9(1), 16-21.

Quinn, P. (1998). *Understanding disability: A lifespan approach*. Thousand Oaks, CA: Sage.

Rapp-Paglicci, L. (2002). Social Exchange Theory in Understanding Human Growth and Development. In J. S. Wodarski, & S. F. Dziegielewki (Eds.), *Human Behavior in the*

Social Environment–Integrating Theory and Evidence-Based Practice (pp. 199-215). New York: Springer Publishing.

Reyes, L. A. (2002). Curriculum Suggestions for Human Behavior. In J. S. Wodarski, & S. F. Dziegielewki (Eds.), *Human Behavior in the Social Environment–Integrating Theory and Evidence-Based Practice* (pp. 295-302). New York: Springer Publishing.

Rothenburg, A. (1975). On anger. In S.A. Pasternak (Ed.), *On violence and victims*. New York: Spectrum.

Salkovskis, P. (1999). Understanding and treating obsessive-compulsive disorder. *Behaviour Research and Therapy*, 37(1), S29-S52.

Salzinger, K. (1969). The place of operant conditioning of verbal behaviors in psychotherapy. In C. Franks (Ed.), *Behavior therapy: Appraisal and status*. New York: McGraw-Hill.

Schmid, T., & Jones, R. (1991). Suspected identity: Identity transformation in a maximum-security prison. *Symbolic Interaction*, 1(40), 415-432.

Schneider, W. J., & Nevid, J. S. (1993). Overcoming math anxiety: A comparison of stress inoculation training and systematic desensitization. *Journal of College Student Development*, 34(4), 283-288.

Schoech, D. (2000). Teaching over the Internet: Results of One Doctoral Course. *Research on Social Work Practice*, 10(4), 467-487.

See, L. A. (1998). Human Behavioral Theory and the African American Experience. *Journal of Human Behavior in the Social Environment*, 1(2/3), 7-29.

Selye, H. (1956). *The stress of life*. Highstown, NJ: McGraw-Hill.

Sherr, M. (2002). Rural Elderly Women: Application of Human Behavior Theory and Issues for Social Work Education. *Journal of Human Behavior in the Social Environment*, 6(4), 47-64.

Skinner, B. F. (1953). *Science and human behavior*. New York: Macmillan.

Skinner, B. F. (1969). *Contingencies of reinforcement*. New York: Appleton-Centure-Crofts.

Smith, C. M., Tindale, R. S., & Dugoni, B. L. (1996). Minority and majority influence in freely interacting groups: Qualitative versus quantitative differences. *British Journal of Social Psychology*, 35(1), 137-149.

Smith, J. F. (1973). Who should do minority research? *Social Casework*, 54(7), 393-397.

Smith, K. D., Leo, C. M., & Maccio, E. M. (2002). Introduction to Human Behavior: Group-Level Variables. In J. S. Wodarski, & S. F. Dziegielewki (Eds.), *Human Behavior in the Social Environment–Integrating Theory and Evidence-Based Practice* (pp. 216-248). New York: Springer Publishing.

Sorensen, G., Lewis, B., & Bishop, R. (1996). Gender, job factors, and coronary heart disease risk. *American Journal of Health Behavior*, 21(1), 3-13.

Spero, M. H. (1982). Programmed Case Material as an Aid in Teaching Ego Psychology: A Methodology for Clinical Social Work Education. *Clinical Social Work Journal*, 10, 190-208.

Stager, S., Chassin, L., & Young, R. (1983). Determinants of self-esteem among labeled adolescents. *Social Psychology Quarterly*, 46, 3-10.

Stinchfield, R. D., & Burlingame, G. M. (1991). Development and use of the directives rating system in group therapy. *Journal of Counseling Psychology*, 39(3), 251-257.

Stocks, J. T., & Freddolino, P. P. (2000). Enhancing Computer-Mediated Teaching Through Interactivity: The Second Iteration of a World Wide Web-Based Graduate Social Work Course. *Research on Social Work Practice*, 10(4), 500-518.

Strathman, A., Gleicher, F., Boninger, D. S., & Edwards, C. S. (1994). The consideration of future consequences: Weighing immediate and distant outcomes of behavior. *Journal of Personality & Social Psychology*, 66(4), 742-752.

Sullivan, M. (2002). Labeling Theory and Human Development. In J. S. Wodarski, & S. F. Dziegielewki (Eds.), *Human Behavior in the Social Environment–Integrating Theory and Evidence-Based Practice* (pp. 110-137). New York: Springer Publishing.

Sutton, C. (1981). Teaching Behavioral Principles to Social Workers: A Comparison of Two Methods of Training. *International Journal of Education for Social Work & Abstracts*, 1, 205-220.

Thyer, B. A. (1996). Guidelines for applying the empirical clinical practice model in social work. *Journal of Applied Social Sciences*, 20(2), 121-127.

Tsuang, M. (2000). Schizophrenia: Genes and environment. *Biological Psychiatry*, 47(3), 210-220.

Vinton, L., & Harrington, P. (1994). An Evaluation of the Use of Videotape in Teaching Empathy. *Journal of Teaching in Social Work*, 9(1/2), 71-84.

Wambach, K. G., Haynes, D. T., & White, B. W. (1999). Practice Guidelines: Rapprochement or Estrangement Between Social Work Practitioners and Researchers. *Research on Social Work Practice*, 9(3), 322-330.

Watson, J. B., & Rayner, R. (1920). Conditioned emotional reaction. *Journal of Experimental Psychology*, 3, 1-14.

Weinert, B. A. (1982). A dialogue for change: Policy, politics, and advocacy. *Administration in Social Work*, 6(2/3), 125-137.

Williams, O. J. (1994). Group work with African American men who batter: Toward more ethnically sensitive practice. *Journal of Comparative Family Studies*, 25(1), 91-104.

Witkin, S. L. (1991). Empirical Clinical Practice: A Critical Analysis. *Social Work*. 36(2), 158-163.

Wodarski, J. S. (1997). *Research methods for clinical social workers*. New York: Springer.

Wodarski, J. S., & Dziegielewki, S. F. (2002). *Human Behavior in the Social Environment–Integrating Theory and Evidence-Based Practice*. New York: Springer Publishing.

Wodarski, J. S., & Feit, M. D. (1994). Applications of reward structures in social group work. *Social Work with Groups*, 17(1/2), 123-142.

Wodarski, J. S., & Feldman, R. A. (1973). The research paradigm: A beginning formulation of process and education objectives. *International Social Work*, 16, 42-48.

Wright, T. L., & Duncan, D. (1986). Attraction to group, group cohesiveness, and individual outcome: A study of training groups. *Small Group Behavior*, 17(4), 487-492.

Yalom, I. D. (1995). *The Theory and Practice of Group Psychotherapy*. New York: HarperCollins.

Ysseldyke, J. E., & Algozzine, B. (1981). Diagnostic classification decision as a function of referral information. *Journal of Special Education*, 15, 429-435.

Zastrow, C. (1999). *The practice of social work* (6th ed.). CA: Brooks-Cole.

APPENDIX 1

Syllabi for Human Behavior in the Social Environment–
Micro/Macro/Mezzo Issues

COURSE-SEQUENCE DESCRIPTION

This two semester course-sequence examines the major social science theories that inform the social work profession's understanding of human behavior in social systems. An ecological/systems framework, together with a developmental approach, is used to provide an interactional understanding of human behavior. The course-sequence opens with an overview of ecological/systems theory, social constructionism, and critical theory with an introduction to the diversity perspective. Social systems are examined across the course sequence, looking at community, organizations, groups, families, and individuals within both traditional and alternative perspectives. Social and economic influences that are addressed include poverty, racism, sexism, and homophobia. Development across the life span is conceptualized as the interplay between nature and nurture where biological and psycho-social risks influence individual resiliency and environmental competence. A biopsychosocial perspective is used throughout the course to inform and examine the interaction between biological, social, psychological, spiritual, and cultural systems. A focus on empirically based theories and knowledge between and among individuals, groups, societies, and economic systems are incorporated. HBSE I examines the life cycle using an ecological perspective from infancy through adolescence. HBSE II continues this examination from young adulthood through senescence. Both units consider the influence of different systems on the health and well-being of the life cycle.

COURSE-SEQUENCE RATIONALE

The content in this course-sequence focuses on human behavior in communities, organizations, groups, families, and life span development in the context of social structures, such as race, ethnicity, social class, and gender roles. Because no one theory is adequate to encompass the human experience, students need to understand the explanatory power of various theories of human behavior within an ecological/systems framework. An ability to both critique and apply theory is a precursor for professional assessments of clients and client situations, as a guide for interventions, and for increasing client empowerment in their environments.

COURSE-SEQUENCE OBJECTIVES

Upon completion of the course-sequence students are expected to be able to:

1. Understand and use a social systems/ecological framework to analyze human systems at different levels of organization from communities to individual;
2. Critique selected social theories from a diversity perspective;
3. Compare historical and traditional perspectives of community with emerging alternative manifestations of community;
4. Demonstrate knowledge of the similarities and differences in various types of family organization and their effects on the life course;
5. Demonstrate knowledge of risk and protective factors in the development of resiliency across the life span;
6. Identify the effects of ethnic, racial, cultural, economic, and gender variables on individuals and families over the life span;
7. Demonstrate knowledge of the interactive influence of biological, psychological, and social factors, including families, groups, organizations, and communities, on human development and behavior;
8. Demonstrate knowledge of the impact of environmental conditions such as class, poverty, oppression, and discrimination on the promotion and inhibition of behavior and development;
9. Demonstrate skill of critiquing evidence-base theories and their applicability for social work practice;
10. Demonstrate knowledge of mezzo-related concerns and the impact it has on individuals and groups.

COURSE ACTIVITIES

1. This activity will be illustrated in class. Over the course of the semester select three empirical-based studies which use any of theoretical

concepts of human development covered in class. Presentations of these articles will address each of these areas:

a. Identify the model(s) used by the authors
b. Identify how well the study conforms to the theories constructs
c. Discuss how well the study describes, explains, and predicts human behavior
d. How does the article address any diversity variables? Any ethical concerns?
e. Discuss what generalizations can be drawn from the selected study
f. Discuss the implications for social work practice
g. If you were to replicate this study, what issues would you address to minimize the problem areas?

APPENDIX 2

Websites Targeting Evidence-Base Practices

Bandolier–Evidence Based Health Care

http://www.jr2.ox.ac.uk/bandolier/

University of Oxford–Centre of Evidence-Based Mental Health

http://cebmh.warne.ox.ac.uk/cebmh/

University of Alberta–Centre for Health Evidence

http://www.cche.net/usersguides/main.asp

Netting the Evidence–Core Library for Evidence Based Practice

http://www.sheffield.ac.uk/~scharr/ir/netting/

University Health Network–Mount Sinai Hospital

http://www.cebm.utoronto.ca/practise/

MedWeb@Emory University–Evidence Based Medicine

http://www.medweb.emory.edu/MedWeb/

BMJ Publishing Group, Royal College of Psychiatrists, & British Psychological Society

http://ebmh.bmjjournals.com/

University of Maryland–Health Sciences and Human Services Library
http://www.hshsl.umaryland.edu/resources/evidence.html
Agency for Healthcare Research and Quality–Evidence Based Practice
http://www.ahcpr.gov/clinic/epcix.htm
University of Washington–Evidence-Based Practice and Guidelines
http://healthlinks.washington.edu/clinical/guidelines.html
State University of New York–Center for Evidence Based Practice
http://www.upstate.edu/fmed/cebp/

Towards a Comprehensive Framework for Understanding the Social Environment: In Search of Theory for Practice

Elizabeth A. Mulroy
Michael J. Austin

SUMMARY. This paper presents a conceptual framework for selecting and organizing concepts of the social environment. It expands upon the traditional Human Behavior and the Social Environment perspectives used in social work curricula in the United States by identifying how a *macro-system* consisting of the intersection of four societal forces (social justice, social problems, social policy, and the political economy) works to influence a *micro-system* of community, organizational, and group dynamics. In this framework, the impact of the macrosystem is mediated by

---

Elizabeth A. Mulroy, PhD, is Associate Professor, School of Social Work, University of Maryland-Baltimore (E-mail: emulroy@ssw.umaryland.edu). Michael J. Austin, PhD, is Professor, School of Social Welfare, University of California-Berkeley (E-mail: mjaustin@uclink.berkeley.edu).

The authors thank Rick Presbury, Livia Munk Davis, and other managers at the Housing Assistance Corporation, Cape Cod, MA for their gracious assistance in facilitating access to the organization as the subject of the case study used in this paper. The authors are grateful to Rino Patti, Paul Ephross, and Jonathan Prince for their thoughtful critiques of the manuscript. The authors also want to acknowledge the able assistance of their doctoral research assistant, Sarah Taylor, who provided them with valuable feedback on this paper.

[Haworth co-indexing entry note]: "Towards a Comprehensive Framework for Understanding the Social Environment: In Search of Theory for Practice." Mulroy, Elizabeth A., and Michael J. Austin. Co-published simultaneously in *Journal of Human Behavior in the Social Environment* (The Haworth Social Work Practice Press, an imprint of The Haworth Press, Inc.) Vol. 10, No. 3, 2004, pp. 25-59; and: *The Conundrum of Human Behavior in the Social Environment* (ed: Marvin D. Feit and John S. Wodarski) The Haworth Social Work Practice Press, an imprint of The Haworth Press, Inc., 2004, pp. 25-59. Single or multiple copies of this article are available for a fee from The Haworth Document Delivery Service [1-800-HAWORTH, 9:00 a.m. - 5:00 p.m. (EST). E-mail address: docdelivery@haworthpress.com].

© 2004 by The Haworth Press, Inc. All rights reserved.
Digital Object Identifier: 10.1300/J137v10n03_02

collective responses of partnerships, alliances, and networks convened to address these forces. The framework is useful for understanding the complexity and uncertainty of the social environment in modern society with specific reference to: (1) how macro-system forces work to shape a constellation of community and organizational concerns, (2) how collective responses that seek solutions can be understood as instruments for achieving meaningful social change, and (3) how micro-systems concepts of structure (stages of development, systems of exchange, and diversity) and process (power and leadership, conflict and change, and integrating mechanisms) can inform practice. *[Article copies available for a fee from The Haworth Document Delivery Service: 1-800-HAWORTH. E-mail address: <docdelivery@haworthpress.com> Website: <http://www.HaworthPress.com> © 2004 by The Haworth Press, Inc. All rights reserved.]*

KEYWORDS. Social environment theory, community theory, collaboration, group dynamics, social justice

The concept of the social environment is important to social workers because it matters *where* and under *what conditions* people live. All people are supported or diminished by the quality and safety of their immediate living environments and the resources, opportunities, and threats to which they are exposed on a daily basis. This aspect of environment is commonly referred to as "community."

We propose that the concept of community has changed in profound ways over the past 30 years and to understand the social environment today one must appreciate the nature of these changes. With renewed attention to the reciprocal relationship between human behavior and the social environment, especially in the Council on Social Work (CSWE) accreditation standards (2001), it is timely to explore these emerging issues in depth. However, before this important task can be fully addressed we need to develop clearer boundaries around the complex nature of the social environment. This is the focus of this paper, with the ultimate goal of promoting further analysis and research on defining the nature of the impact of the social environment on human behavior, and the impact of human behavior on the social environment. The specification of this reciprocal relationship is a much larger agenda that is beyond the scope of this analysis.

The dynamics of community change occurred in what Warren (1978) called the *micro-system* and the *macro-system*. We make a distinction between the practice terminology of micro (clinical work with individuals), mezzo (interventions with groups and families), and macro (interventions related to community practice, management practice, and policy practice) and our social science terms of macro-systems and micro-systems. Local communities, in Warren's paradigm, comprise the micro-system in which local community-based organizations, once imbued with independent power and influence, no longer achieve their purposes with local resources alone. The micro-system has been social work's traditional focal area of community practice (Netting, Kettner, & McMurtry, 1993; Hardcastle, Wenocur, & Powers, 1997; Rothman, Erlich, & Tropman, 2001) as well as the traditional focal area of the social environment in HB&SE curricula (Taylor, Austin, & Mulroy, 2004). However, macro- system changes such as the global economy and rapid technological change contributed to a restructuring of urban America, a phenomenon that typically occurred beyond the influence or control of local communities and their neighborhoods (Mier & Giloth, 1993). Local communities, however, have horizontal linkages to other organizations in the local micro-system and vertical linkages to the macro-system. In addition to understanding the nature of the micro and macro systems, it is important to understand the ways in which vertical links shape, facilitate, and constrain community, organizational, and group dynamics (Warren, 1978).

The conceptualization of the social environment in terms of macro- and micro-systems involves an exploration of the following questions: (1) What is the role of social justice in facilitating one's understanding of the social environment? (2) How do social problems and public policies continuously impact communities in which organizations are located? (3) How is the social environment linked with the physical environment and what are the impacts on community well-being and inter-organizational relations? and (4) How do community factors and relationships that are external to an organization impact groups and organizations? Each of these questions served as a guide for the development of a comprehensive framework for understanding the key concepts inherent in the construct of the social environment.

A purpose of this article is to identify the properties of the macro-system that influence the micro-system. While it is acknowledged that the larger framework includes human behavior and the social environment, this article focuses on a clarification of the concept of the social environment, an area that has not received much attention from social work scholars. First, we present a conceptual framework in Figure 1 that seeks to capture the impact of the macro perspective of the social environment on local conditions and dynamics. Four societal level forces are identified and will be discussed. They are social justice, social problems, social policies, and the political economy. Then we analyze the ways in which they link and interact, suggesting the direct influences of societal forces on local-level conditions and dynamics. We propose that embedded in the social environment are *collective responses* that serve as intermediary mechanisms between the macro and micro-systems. These responses involve cooperation and/or collaboration among diverse parties who seek solutions to vexing societal issues and movement forward toward social change through problem solving. Gray (1989) suggests that a theory of collaboration is dynamic and process-oriented; it is a negotiated order that allows people affected by environmental turbulence and uncertainty to respond collectively. This theory postulates that collaboration is a temporary and emergent organization form. It accommodates differing organizational interests, and is a vehicle for action learning.

The macro-systems elements in the social environment are then examined from the micro-system perspective. We begin this section by introducing a case vignette of the Housing Assistance Corporation, a community-based nonprofit organization that is attempting to find a permanent solution to homelessness in order to better serve homeless individuals and families while also helping to build a healthy, caring community for all residents. The core issues of the case are presented,

FIGURE 1. Macro Perspective of the Social Environment: Influences of Societal Level Macro-Systems Forces on Local Micro-Systems Conditions and Dynamics

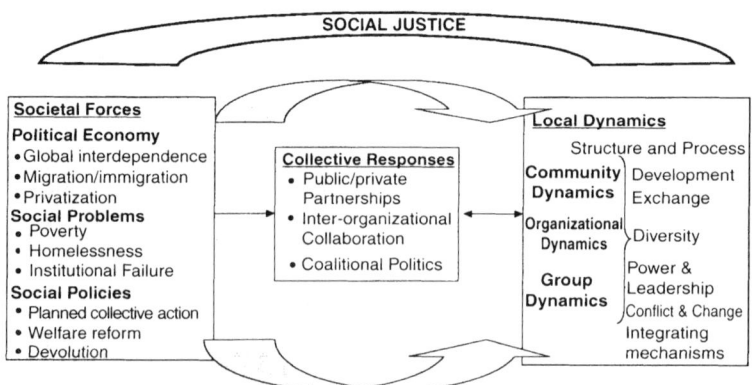

followed by questions for the reader that draw implications of macro societal forces for the micro-system. We return to the case again at the conclusion of the article.

The concepts of structure and process are used to explain the micro-systems of community neighborhoods, organizations, and group activity as well as the inter-relationships between these three sectors using major organizing concepts. Finally, we draw conclusions relative to our search for key concepts related to the social environment and how they might inform social work practice and research. To do this we return to a discussion of the case vignette of the Housing Assistance Corporation using the main concepts introduced throughout the article. Because the elements of the macro- and micro-systems are derived from many fields, we draw from a multi-disciplinary literature. Selected classic works from the 1960s and 1970s are used from urban theory, community theory, and organizational theory where, given current conditions, they demonstrated remarkable prescience.

THE MACRO-SYSTEM PERSPECTIVE

About 30 years ago, noted scholar Anthony Downs wrote in his book *Urban Problems and Prospects*

> Technical and economic factors, plus cultural and spiritual ones, are shifting much more rapidly than our legal and social institutions. The result is an escalation of general tensions and conflicts, and great pressure for major alterations in even the most basic institutions. . . . By *institutions* I mean established laws and organizational structures, their rules, their interrelations, and the entrenched patterns of behavior built around them. (1973, p. 1)

Downs argued that to address urban problems–including environmental pollution, high crime rates, hunger, poverty, racism, poor housing, and poor education–we would need bold initiatives, institutional change, and a political approach to policy analysis requiring a consideration of the *redistributive* impacts of any policy proposals.

How can practitioners understand the social environment from this macrosystem perspective? A point of departure is to understand that four societal forces–social justice, social problems, social policies, and the political economy–are powerful societal forces with characteristics that influence local dynamics in profound ways.

Understanding Societal Forces: Social Justice, Social Problems, Social Policies, and the Political Economy

1. Social Justice. The principles of social justice have long been associated with the mission of the social work profession. The recent focus on violence, oppression, and trauma–be it in war-torn Iraq, gay-bashing youth cultures, or drug-dealing street corners in poor urban neighborhoods–has raised renewed interest and concern in the profession and in the larger society about social justice (Marsh, 2003; Bailey, 2003; Fields, 2003). Concepts of social justice are often framed by political ideologies and religious beliefs.

The overall construct of social justice can be viewed from individual, institutional, and geographic perspectives. Solomon (1995) suggests that justice is not a utopian plan for the perfect society but a personal, individual and a collective sense of responsibility. From this perspective, social justice operates from the bottom up, grounded in individual experience and emotion that results in a person's *moral sensibility*, or personal sense of outrage in the face of real human misery. Solomon suggests that justice, as a natural sentiment, offers an inborn sense of our connectedness to others, a mutual concern, and shared interests. This natural feeling may unleash compassion for the larger community or commonwealth (1995; 153-172). This sense of justice requires the recognition of basic needs and therefore basic rights, as intrinsically legitimate demands that are binding on anyone who is able to help. David Gil (1998) suggests that social justice is the absence of injustice and oppression. Oppression is seen as a mode of human relations that involves exploitation, marginalization, powerlessness, cultural imperialism, and violence between social groups and classes and globally between societies (Gil, 1998; Van Soest & Garcia, 2003).

Moral philosopher John Rawls (1971) argues that (social) justice means 'fairness . . .': 'the principle subject of justice is the basic structure of society . . . the way in which the major social institutions distribute fundamental rights and duties and determine the division of advantages from *social* cooperation . . .' (Rawls, 1971, as quoted in Craig, 2002, p. 669; italics in original). Social justice, according to Longres and Scanlon (2001), has two dimensions. One is distributive justice that refers to the way economic and social goods and services are distributed in a society. The other is relational justice that refers to the decision making processes and relationships between dominant and subordinate groups that affect the decisions made about the distribution of goods and services (p. 448).

A key question posed by urban theorist David Harvey is this: What is being distributed, and to whom is it being distributed it? He suggests that the essence of social justice is embodied in three criteria: need, contribution to the common good, and merit. He introduces *territorial social justice*, a geographic-based concept that envisions (1) a distribution of income that takes individual need into account with extra resources allocated to overcome special difficulties stemming from the physical and social environment, and (2) mechanisms (institutional, organizational, political, and economic) that help to level the geographic playing field so that the prospects for disadvantaged geographic areas are as great as they possibly can be (Harvey, 1973, 116-117).

British social work scholar Gary Craig is asking similar questions (2002). He summarizes a view of social justice that synthesizes individual, institutional, and territorial perspectives while incorporating diversity and the values of dignity, equality of outcomes, and participation. Social justice is

> ... A framework of political objectives, pursued through social, economic, environmental, and political policies, based on an acceptance of difference and diversity, and informed by values concerned with:
>
> - achieving fairness, and equality of outcomes and treatment;
> - recognizing the dignity and equal worth and encouraging the self-esteem of all;
> - the meeting of basic needs;
> - maximizing the reduction of inequalities in wealth, income, and life chances; and
> - the participation of all, including the most disadvantaged. (Craig, 2002, 671-672)

If the principle subject of social justice is the structure of society, as Rawls suggests, then its relation to social problems, social policies, and the political economy becomes a central theme in understanding the complexity of the social environment, and in crafting practice solutions that address systemic oppression and injustice.

2. Social Problems. The definition of what constitutes a social problem is fundamentally a framing issue; social conditions become social problems when society decides they should be improved (Julian, 1977). For a social problem to exist, there needs to be (1) objective, documented evidence of a social condition (e.g., increasing numbers of persons without shelter and a place to live, or increasing numbers of children who are abused or neglected), and (2) subjective evidence or belief that the social problem (e.g., "homelessness" or "child maltreatment") should be remedied or changed. One of the most pervasive and intractable social problems is poverty (Healy, 2001). Poverty is the root cause of most other social problems such as poor maternal and child health, illiteracy, substance abuse, hunger, the spread of AIDS, and homelessness.

The relationship between poverty in the United States and poverty around the world is a complex phenomenon. According to the United Nations Development Program (1996) . . . "poverty is no longer contained within national boundaries. It has become globalized. It travels across borders, without a passport, in the form of drugs, diseases, pollution, migration, terrorism, and political instability" (quoted in Healy, 2001, p. 119). The poorest are mostly women and their children.

There are four aspects of framing social problems that merit discussion. First, social problems are typically difficult to define and classify. For example, is substance abuse a physical problem, a mental problem, or is it anti-social behavior (Jansson, 1994)? Second, a series of premises and assumptions are made as to what constitutes a social problem. A certain social structure and culture can induce people to conform, but can also cause some people to deviate. The assessment of a social condition is based on patterns of behavior, religious beliefs, political ideologies, and perceptions based on an overall view of the world. Therefore the background of groups involved and the environments from which they come are significant factors in identifying and defining a particular social problem (Julian, 1977; 1-8).

Third, the physical location for problem definition and resolution has changed. Historically community leaders expected to solve their own community's social problems, and local control was a rallying cry. But today, the relationship between urban problems as earlier defined by Downs (1973) and social problems are blurred. Unemployment and local economic development, for example, are affected by national economic conditions, by interdependencies that now include the global nature of information technology and the transnational flow of capital and of jobs, as well as changing political perceptions and paradigms of causality. These vertical linkages with the macro-systems affect many types of local micro-systems in areas such as poverty, homelessness, and substance abuse and have a profound impact on creating community-based solutions.

Fourth, social problems provide a major challenge to American institutions. Institutions can be part of the problem and/or part of the solution. *Institutional failures* can exacerbate or create new social problems. Increased homelessness, for example, creates a need for responsive public housing institutions and shelter/service arrangements. Yet the public policy response–the temporary shelter system–has neither fostered independence nor solved homelessness. Federal housing policy as well as many state and county public agencies and their for-profit and nonprofit contractors have come under scrutiny for failing to provide housing as a basic human right (Smizik & Stone, 1988; Wolch & Dear, 1993). Some common examples of institutional failures in the human services area to address social problems include:

- Fragmentation: Barriers among multiple, uncoordinated programs
- Discontinuity: Clients cannot obtain consistent, accessible services over time
- Lack of access: Barriers to service use at different sites
- Discrimination: Service providers hostile or indifferent to specific kinds of clients
- "Creaming": Providers intentionally seek out clients who are easier to serve
- Wastage: Inefficient service provision by organizations to the same beneficiaries
- Lack of outreach: Providers make little effort to recruit persons who do not currently use services
- Overburdened staff: Understaffed departments where employees are asked to perform tasks for which they have little training
- Lack of cultural sensitivity: Little effort made by providers to match services with cultural perspective of consumers (Jansson, 1994; 4-6).

These also represent failures in the implementation of social policies, policies that were originally enacted to alleviate or ameliorate social problems.

3. Social Policies. A *social policy is a collective strategy to address social problems* such as poverty, mental illness, or hunger (Jansson, 1994, p. 4, italics in original). We collectively respond to social problems and to people who are socially excluded by enacting social policies. Social policy in the United States is a government activity at federal, state, and local levels intended to enhance people's welfare through a variety of means: The creation of social service programs, the use of statutory regulation, and the tax system (Midgley, 2000). The courts also play a major role in social policy formation by interpreting government legislation and by examining constitutional issues when it decides cases that concern the welfare of individuals and of certain groups. Social policies also address institutional failures in the social service delivery system when barriers to program implementation arise. There may be a need to change a social policy by (1) amending original legislation, (2) issuing new government regulations, (3) changing the budget that funded the program, (4) or changing policy at specific program sites to better meet local needs (Jansson, 1994).

For example, The Personal Responsibility and Work Opportunity Reconciliation Act of 1996 ended the entitlement to public assistance for very poor people. As "welfare reform" it has large-scale impacts not only on the targeted beneficiaries but on existing social institutions, particularly those federal, state, and county public agencies mandated to implement it, and their for-profit and local-serving nonprofit vendors.

While child abuse and neglect, poor health, and poverty seem clear examples of social problems that require a social policy response, what actually constitutes a social policy as opposed to another kind of policy such as economic or environmental is less clear. Some scholars in the field argue that specific policies regarding housing, taxes, job training, and economic development become social policies whenever they influence or exacerbate social problems (Jansson, 1994). Therefore social policies can range from high-level national legislative policies to local policies that affect neighborhoods where intransigent social problems such as homelessness actually exist.

The collective action dimension of social policy lends itself to controversy. Values and experience frame our perspectives on social problems that result in a range of conservative, liberal, and radical perspectives within the policy debate. In the final analysis, policy makers typically express their policy priorities based on perceived constituent preferences. Concerned with recent trends in social policy, a prominent social reformer like Alvin Schorr (1997) calls on individuals to take a stand based on their deepest convictions. Underscoring the principles of social justice discussed earlier he calls for egalitarianism, sympathy and respect for the underdog, a sense of community and belief in the need for community building, and a view that government should be of the people and owes them empathy and responsiveness. He writes:

> It has been my view that, just as our values create our institutions, in turn our institutions and social structures *create* our values.

Thus, social security *created* the modern concept of retirement, and French children's allowances undergird the devotion of the French to children. Even apart from believing that if we created our institutions the values would follow, I rarely wrote about values per se because it seemed hard to do without sounding pious or vague. However, the pervasive greed that has settled upon Americans is a thing in itself now, making it almost irrelevant to argue for true community-centered policies. So I place first in this matter of taking a stand the examination and assertion of one's deepest principles and an attempt to take back the policy debate from our grossest social predators and their attendant rationalizers and flacks. However, economic and institutional developments constrain whether we can find our way back to a decent society. (Schorr, 1997, pp. 185-186)

While social problems and social policies are visible manifestations that can be documented in the Congressional Record economic and institutional developments play out in the global political economy, an invisible domain of activity.

4. Political Economy. Political economy is the intersection of events and decisions in a politically organized community that has economic implications and political considerations (Feagin, 1998; Lefebrvre, 1991). The concept of a political economy is based on the premise that the structure and evolution of any society depends principally on that society's dominant mode of economic production. Social problems, therefore, have economic roots, and need to be understood as symptoms of institutional causes driven principally by economic forces in the environment. Warren (1978) suggests that anyone who has interest in the economic viability of local communities must turn to the economics of the macro-system. Therefore we will now use a political economy perspective as a way to identify and analyze the presence of vertical links in the macro-system and their relationship to local community activity in the micro-system.

Of the many factors in the macro-system that affect local communities we chose to illustrate urban restructuring, global interdependencies, and privatization because of their relevance to the specific social problems and social policies discussed above. The large arrows in Figure 1 depict the direct linkages between all of these societal forces and local-level dynamics.

First, Gottdiener, and Pickvance (1993) suggest that since the 1970s, *urban restructuring* has transformed urban America. One aspect is the restructuring of the economic base from industrial production to high technology manufacturing and information processing. The other is demographic, and includes the massive shift in population as middle-class child-rearing families moved out of cities to the suburbs and new immigrant groups moved in. The social life of city neighborhoods changed with the infusion of diverse racial, cultural, and ethnic newcomers. By the 1980s and 1990s the impacts of such *urban restructuring* found *cities* pitted against each other in the fight for national government funds. Local politics changed to reflect the new resident demographics, culture, conflicts, and power. Some cities experienced periods of economic turnaround and renewal, periods that were followed most recently by fiscal crisis at both state and city levels (Katz, 2000; Gottdiener & Pickvance, 1993).

In an analysis of the U.S. Census for 2000, Frey (2002) found that traditional concepts of urban/suburban/rural communities no longer hold. Instead, new regional divisions have emerged across America shaped by very different immigration and domestic migration flows. These population patterns are creating three new regions, each with its own cultural and demographic personality: the "New Sunbelt" states (primarily in the South), an increasingly diverse "Melting Pot" states (like California, New York, Texas, Florida, Illinois, and New Jersey), and the "Aging, Slow-Growing Heartland" states (primarily in the Midwest).

Second, the global economy and a myriad of *global interdependencies* emerged with serious social welfare implications. Three examples include the worldwide labor pool, migration, and immigration discussed above, and global spread of HIV/AIDS. According to Healy (2001), the flaws of the global economy include long-term unemployment, labor insecurity, debt, and low-incomes; all with negative impacts on the human condition felt not only in the United States but also worldwide. Economic interdependencies are created through world trade, currency regulations, foreign aid, and lending patterns. Working on the principle of "economies of scale," multinational corporations grow even bigger through mergers and acquisitions. In the last three years more than $1.5 trillion worth of companies changed hands (Henry, Der Hovanesian, & Foust, 2003). Products are then produced through complex arrangements in many different countries, as labor is sought at the most inexpensive source (e.g., India, China, Ireland, or Haiti).

Third, *privatization* is a related trend that has had dramatic impacts on the delivery of health and social services at state, county, and neighborhood levels. Over several decades, and under both republican and democratic political regimes, the funding and delivery of social welfare services shifted from the public sector to a reliance on private nonprofit and for-profit organizations. The privatization of health and human services (such as managed care) emphasizes business principles of accountability and efficiency outcomes. Research conducted by Fabricant and Fisher (2002) and Wolch (1990) suggests that small, community-based nonprofit organizations with a clear concept of the public interest and progressive, social change missions targeted to serve very low-income populations have been financially hard-hit under privatization. These social change organizations are unlikely competitors for state and county contracts against large nonprofit and for-profit organizations, particularly those with extensive contacts with the state, and the capability to offer large public bureaucracies a variety of services to meet a range of state or county administrative and service needs.

Gibelman and Demone (2002) examined privatization of health and human services from a social justice perspective and found equity implications along the following dimensions: access, cost, continuity, and quality of care. They pose several important questions: Are nonprofits being priced out of existence? What is the extent to which for-profits focus on some social problems and not others? To what extent does the profit motive affect the type and quality of services offered? To what extent does the profit motive compromise the public interest and human well-being? From the perspective of political economy the role of the state is critically important to the generation of equitable solutions. Therefore, as Schorr (1997) suggests, research, policy analysis, and advocacy need to be conducted through the lens of social justice in order to influence the social policy debate.

However, the full effects of the societal forces discussed above can be deeply felt by citizens and practitioners across regions, in counties, cities, and in neighborhoods. Diverse constituencies have forged new cooperative and collaborative relationships to address the impacts of these macro-systems forces. The nature of these collective responses is examined next.

Collective Responses as Mediating Structures

Collective responses are formal and informal governance structures designed to respond to and find solutions for changing environmental conditions and social problems situated in larger social systems. During the 1980s and throughout the 1990s local citizens and professionals came to realize that "places have relationships and connections to other places that cannot be ignored" (Katz, 2000, p. 3). It was evident that social problems were interrelated, had long histories of policy initiatives and failures, and their domains intersected often across jurisdictional boundaries. By the 1950s and 1960s large public housing projects for the poor, for example, were concentrated and isolated in particular inner-city neighborhoods. This was not necessarily the intended outcome of housing policy but was more the result of well-organized citizen resistance to public housing in middle-income neighborhoods and the pressure of urban politics on pliant housing bureaucracies (Meehan, 1979). Later, coalitions of housing advocates who wanted to unravel the complexity and disperse the poor linked public housing decisions with those of public schools, transportation, and jobs not only in the city but in surrounding suburbs. In another example, managers in human service agencies began to appreciate that one agency alone did not have the resources or expertise to address the complexity of problems faced by troubled clients. Human service organizations recognized that it would take several agencies working together as partners (including those outside a "target" neighborhood) to assist the increasing number of families beset with multiple problems who lived in communities beset with an increasing level of violence and other environmental stressors (Mulroy, 2003). Thus, the concept of community has expanded. The focal point will increasingly be the metropolitan region, though attention will continue to focus on cities, counties, towns, and neighborhoods.

Leadership was sought to build new social relationships and institutions capable of solving social problems for these diverse forms of community (Mier & Giloth, 1993). Gray (1989) contends that such leadership will benefit from cooperative and collaborative processes. She proposes multiple designs that differ according to two factors: (1) the motivating factors of the problem under consideration, and (2) the intended outcomes. For example, a motivating factor could be either to advance a shared vision or to resolve a conflict. The intended outcome could be either to exchange information or to formalize a joint agreement. These factors determine the type of collective response suitable to the situation (Gray, 1989). Research suggests that collective responses may produce positive and/or negative unintended consequences. To illustrate the construct of collective responses we have identified public/private partnerships, inter-organizational service networks, and coalitional politics as examples.

Public/Private/Partnerships. For the past several decades, mayors of large and small cities, members of County Councils, and elected state officials confronted reduced federal support, population loss, and a declining local revenue base. They turned to "captains" of industry as partners with a presumed shared vision to revitalize sagging economies. Over time, these public/private partnerships emerged as business coalitions, often with nonprofit tax status, and as elite driving forces in regional economies. Some corporate partners had a clear concept of the public interest and committed resources and time to local economic development and revitalization projects. Other partners with business affiliations in the global economy were less concerned with local issues. While business investment and a large-view perspective continue to be important factors in civic problem solving, Kanter (2000) found that such partnerships were often shadow governments. Their business interests influenced public decision making, and in the end, failed to account for local jurisdictional differences such as the diverse needs and assets of local towns, cities, or counties. This raised the question of whether such partnerships were in fact operating in the "public interest" since they did not account for geographic disparities based on race and economic segregation, lack of affordable housing, inadequate public transit systems out of central cities to places of employment, or the impact on failing inner city public schools. Some partnerships located new employment opportunities in suburban or even farther out in "exurban" areas that are far removed from a city's struggling urban core.

Inter-Organizational Service Networks. Based on organization theory, inter-organizational service networks are complex structures in which several social agencies work together as equal partners on two levels–administratively, and on the front lines of service delivery. Both levels embrace a team-oriented, participatory management style to jointly plan for and implement a range of services and activities to which each agency contributes a part. Successful networks share a common vision based on a social justice element (such as the reduction of homelessness or child abuse and neglect), agree upon methods to achieve the desired ends, share risks and rewards, and formalize the relationship with joint agreements (Adams & Nelson, 1998; Mulroy, 1997). Service networks may operate at state, county, and local neighborhood levels. They may be mandated by state regulations to improve service integration and increase resources for intended beneficiaries. Participants are integral to larger community building and social development processes when working with residents in a local neighborhood in a community-based network. Inter-organizational service networks, however, are not without conflicts since not all collective responses are motivated by the desire to advance a shared vision as the next example illustrates.

Coalitional Politics. The desire to resolve conflict over a controversial issue may also motivate a collective response, particularly when multiple stakeholder groups are involved and the power dynamics among the groups range from low to high. Some examples include deciding on a site for a homeless shelter, a methadone treatment facility, or a residential group home for persons exiting prison.

Since this approach is based on power sharing, one critical issue is to find a way to agree on *solutions*. The challenges are complex. For example, land use planning decision structures responsible for zoning may be spread across a region—a wide geographic area that may include several legislative districts, neighborhoods, town councils, and land use commissions. Similarly, the NIMBY (not in my backyard) phenomenon catalyzes a number of groups to participate, and "stakeholders who are organized enough to have capacity will be included" (Gray, 1989, p. 120). Therefore coalitional politics acknowledges the power differential among stakeholder groups; it seeks a negotiated settlement as the final outcome while planning for the success of a range of interim outcomes that make the final outcome possible. For example, grass roots community organizing is used prior to collaboration to prepare "voiceless" groups to acquire an empowered position and sense of self to participate in issue framing, direction setting, and implementation (Gray, 1989). Issue advocacy is used at the outset to convene public meetings that guarantee widespread participation of all parties thought to have a stakeholder interest in the issue, including political office holders and beneficiaries. Then the process itself must be mediated. Both public and private sector leaders are now turning to executives of nonprofit organizations for leadership in mediating complex multiparty disputes because they are perceived to be neutral, ethical, and fair (Kanter, 2000). Coalitional politics assumes that the issues, when eventually understood and appreciated by all parties as community-owned problems, have the potential to be settled through negotiation; only then can meaningful social change be achieved. As Gray (1989) suggests, "collaboration is a process through which parties who see different aspects of a problem can constructively explore their differences and search for solutions that go beyond their own limited vision of what is possible" (p. 5).

In sum, this section has defined properties of the macro-system (social justice, social problems, social policies, the political economy, and collective responses) as depicted in our model (Figure 1), then analyzed some of the ways they intersect and contribute to the vastness and complexity of the social environment. The arrows in Figure 1 suggest that local level dynamics are influenced by two sets of forces. The first set of forces comes directly from social problems, social policies, and the political economy (as depicted by the large arrows). The second set comes indirectly from the effects of collective responses–themselves a reaction to societal forces (see small arrow). The two-way arrow between collective responses and local dynamics in Figure 1 suggests that collective responses are intermediary mechanisms with interactive properties. That is, local citizens, practitioners, business interests, and decision makers influence the form and outcome of collective responses, and the nature of the responses in turn influence local dynamics. Social justice in Figure 1 is shown as an overarching perspective with the potential to influence all elements–societal forces, collective responses, and local dynamics. The next section examines the micro-system of local communities, organizations, and group dynamics and the linkages to the macro-system.

THE MICRO-SYSTEM PERSPECTIVE

The substance of the model described above is clearly consequential for local institutions. If certain macro-system forces perpetuate injustice, fail to address social problems effectively, and funded policies and collective responses themselves generate negative social consequences, then local institutions and the populations they serve will likely suffer. Conversely, local institutions may analyze macro forces and respond proactively with innovative solutions. These may draw together a wide range of horizontal linkages based on local community and institutional support, and searching out vertical ties that bring new resources into the locality. To illustrate these points we present a case vignette (Figure 2) of the Housing Assistance Corporation.

After twenty years of providing shelters and services to homeless individuals and families the community-based nonprofit organization decided to help its many clients in another way. It reframed the problem of homelessness and moved to a social strategy that systemically addressed the problem of homelessness as a community and a societal problem. The questions posed in Figure 2 are intended to assist in the examination of the macro-system forces on the micro-system of the local community, the substance of the section that follows.

FIGURE 2. The Housing Assistance Corporation Responds to Homelessness

The Housing Assistance Corporation (HAC) is a regional nonprofit organization on Cape Cod, MA that opened its doors in 1974 in response to seasonal shifts in the tourist-dependent economy that helped create housing problems and homelessness. Cape demographics indicate a mix of wealthy and middle-income people as well as a very diverse population of low-income and disadvantaged persons needing affordable housing. Federal and state housing policies drastically reduced funds for affordable housing nationally. Renters locked out of urban housing markets migrated to the Cape in search of affordable housing. But as growth and development increased across the region in which the Cape is a part, local housing prices soared. A service and a seasonal tourist economy bring in low-wage workers who cannot afford a place to live.

The agency's mission is to promote and implement the right of all people on Cape Cod and the islands (Martha's Vineyard and Nantucket) to occupy safe and affordable housing. Supported with diversified funding from public and private sources, and an active 30-person Board of Directors, the agency served more than 5,000 people in 2001. Included in its eight program areas are six service-intensive shelters serving homeless single persons, parents with children, and persons with addictions.

Using social justice and community building as the core principles of its mission, the organization re-framed the problem of homelessness from an issue facing individuals to a problem facing the community. Several years ago, staff began to recognize that shelters tend to create dependency and do not necessarily address the social problem of homelessness. One program manager (with an MSW) suggested the need for a peaceful setting where disadvantaged people come together as members of a real community—a place to belong—with apartments for which they pay rent, educational and vocational training, and work. The concept, called Dana's Fields, is based on the belief that we all need a stable foundation on which to build our lives, and we are all healthier when we are part of a strong and loving community, rather than excluded and isolated. It is a relationship-based program (not a treatment program) designed to turn around individual lives, create a community built on acceptance and compassion, and address institutional barriers in the housing market that have accelerated the slide into homelessness for vulnerable people.

Staff sought to interpret the philosophy of Dana's Fields to diverse stakeholder groups in order to create a more comprehensive appreciation of the problem of homelessness than any one of the groups could envision alone. Support for the project was gathered through community outreach, including convening public meetings, presentations before regional planning and zoning boards, civic and economic development groups, resistive NIMBY (not in my backyard) groups and their attorneys, and national print and television media. Over time, the needed financial capital was raised to purchase and develop a 46-acre working farm to include 60 units of affordable housing, training programs, and community-use amenities. Ten years after HAC initiated its plan it finally received the all-important land use approval (with conditions) from the local Zoning Board of Appeals that permits ground to be broken for development.

Questions

1. How do key concepts about social justice help to explain (a) the origins and evolution of HAC, and (b) the attainment of community support for Dana's Fields?
2. How does an understanding of the nature of social problems help to explain the sources of homelessness?
3. In what ways does this case identify the range and impact of public policy decisions from national, state, to local levels that affect the problem of homelessness?
4. How can homelessness be explained as both a political and economic problem?
5. What factors can be identified to explain a collective response to homelessness in urbanizing America?

6. What aspects of the Cape Cod community structure (stages of development, systems of exchange, and diversity) and process (power and leadership, conflict and change, and integrating mechanisms) can explain the responsiveness to the problem of homelessness?

7. What aspects of HAC's organizational structure and process can explain its ability to persist in its development of comprehensive services for the homeless?

8. What aspects of group dynamics (structure and process) helped the Cape Cod community and HAC respond to homelessness through the collaboration of citizens and agency personnel?

Understanding the Micro-Systems of the Social Environment: Communities, Groups, and Organizations

There are a set of concepts that provide a framework for understanding the social environment from a micro-systems perspective. As noted earlier, the macro-systems perspectives include the nature of a social problem that, in turn, raises social justice issues and can ultimately lead to the proposal and enactment of social policies. These policies are often implemented at the local level through city or county government as well as by nonprofit and for-profit provider organizations that all comprise a community of organizations. Their inter-organizational network may reflect an array of integrated and/or fragmented service delivery relationships. These relationships include contracted services with shared responsibilities for financing and client services, co-located services with shared responsibility for maintaining access to client services, and integrated services with shared responsibility for promoting the availability of client services (e.g., one-stop shopping). All of these relationships call upon an understanding of the micro-systems perspective of the social environment, namely, the nature of community at the neighborhood level, the nature of community-based human service organizations, and the dynamics of group behavior that underlie citizen involvement in neighborhoods as well as staff involvement inside and outside human service organizations.

Structure and Process

The two most all-encompassing concepts needed to understand communities, groups, and organizations at the local or neighborhood level are *structure* and *process*. Structure refers, in this context, to the arrangement and mutual relationship of the constituent parts to the whole (Brown, 1993). Process is defined, for this discussion, as a continuous series of actions, events, or changes that are directed toward some end and/or performed in a specific manner (Brown, 1993). In essence, how are community neighborhoods and organizations structured? How do groups of citizens and staff behave amongst themselves and with each other? These are critical questions for understanding the social environment of community neighborhoods and organizations that seek to meet the needs of its residents or clients. These community organizations can include public schools, neighborhood service centers, places of worship, child care agencies, senior centers, group homes, women's shelters, and neighborhood health clinics.

Community Neighborhoods: The structure of a neighborhood includes both formal and informal organizations and associations. These could include an informal network of local clergy, an association of neighborhood merchants, a neighborhood after-school program, or a neighborhood substation for the police and fire department. These are all part of the formal and informal structure of a neighborhood community. The concept of structure can be used to identify and assess the processes that underlie a neighborhood's horizontal and vertical relationships (Warren, 1978). For example, the horizontal dimension of process dynamics might include regular neighborhood meetings between the clergy, police, school principals, and service center director. The vertical dimension could include the maintenance of relationships between the neighborhood and the larger community (e.g., city, county, or region). Examples of the vertical dimension include organizational relationships with the county social service and public health departments, school districts, non-profit organizations serving the region, and city police and fire departments. These horizontal and vertical relationships provide another perspective on the vitality of a neighborhood community.

One of the process concepts applicable to a neighborhood community involves community competence (Fellin, 2001, p. 70), namely, the capacity of the neighborhood residents and service providers to engage in a process of identifying community needs, coordinating services, and/or facilitating problem-solving related to community concerns or resolving conflicts.

Community-Based Organizations: Just like neighborhood communities, the concepts of structure and process can also inform our understanding of organizations. For example, all human service organizations have a service mission or purpose. Within such a mission, they can be characterized as primarily people processing, people sustaining, or people changing (Hasenfeld, 1983, p. 5). *People processing* organizations are structured to make sure that those who are eligible for benefits (e.g., Food Stamps, immunizations, etc.) are processed in an effective and efficient manner. *People sustaining* organizations are designed to provide a level of care that is high enough to help individuals and/or families attain self-sufficiency (e.g., group homes, service centers, etc.). *People changing* organizations are structured in a way to provide services that help individuals grow and thrive in their community (e.g., schools, mental health and substance abuse services, etc.).

In addition to the structure of the organization influencing its internal processes, organizations must also contend with their external environment. Examples of the environment that have direct bearing on their neighborhood location could be accessible bus routes or well-established referral relationships with other related organizations. The task environment of an agency can be defined in terms of community involvement (client advisory committees and agency boards of directors), sources of funding (city/county government, United Way, etc.), and political support (elected officials, opinion leaders, and philanthropic funds).

Groups in Communities and Organizations: In addition to the community and organizational dimensions of the social environment, the concepts of structure and process also have relevance for understanding groups that operate within the social environment. The questions about group structure in a neighborhood might be: How are neighborhood groups organized (by blocks or shared concerns)? What are the patterns of communications between neighborhood groups and within groups? Similarly, group process concepts focus on the array of systems and behaviors demonstrated by group members (Patton & Downs, 2003). The questions about neighborhood group processes might include: How are leaders identified? How invested are members in their neighborhood groups? Are the behaviors of group members focused primarily on neighborhood improvement projects or on advocacy efforts focused on city hall?

These same group structure and process concepts can be applied to a neighborhood organization, whether it is the staff of an agency or its board members. How are staff members organized (organization chart, labor-management agreement)? How is the board structured (15 members meeting frequently vs. 60 members meeting infrequently or active use of standing vs. ad hoc committees)? In addition to the structural dimensions, it is important to note the process or group dynamics dimensions. What role do staff members play in organizational decision-making? Are there regularly scheduled staff meetings? Who leads them?

What is the nature of inter-disciplinary collaboration (e.g., neighborhood health clinic staffed by many disciplines)? What is the nature of teamwork and problem-solving between staff representatives and neighborhood client advisory groups? All these questions illustrate the centrality of understanding group processes inside and outside a human service organization.

As noted in Figure 3, the concepts of structure and process are primary elements in fostering an understanding of the social environment that includes neighborhood communities, organizations and groups. These key concepts are also connected to a set of related concepts that elaborate or "drill down deeper" to understand the complexity of structure and process. For example, central to the concept of structure and process are the concepts of *development*, *exchange*, and *diversity*. Each of these is described in the next section.

FIGURE 3. The Concepts of Structure and Process for Understanding the Micro-Systems of the Social Environment

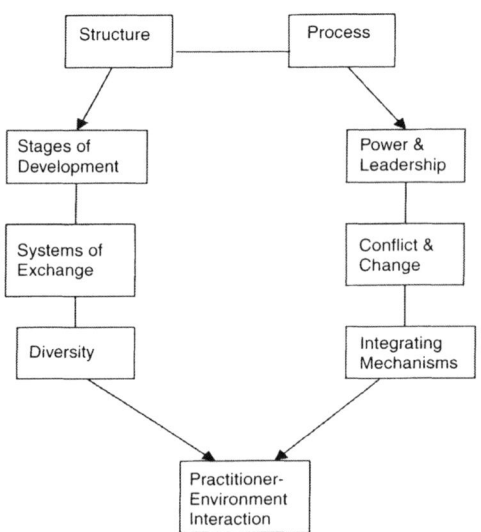

ELEMENTS OF STRUCTURE

Stages of Development

The term "stages of development" refers to the location of the community, group and organization along a continuum of time and evolution. For example, such a continuum is important for understanding the social environment of a community neighborhood in terms of its stability over time or its changing nature (improving or declining). The same stage of development continuum applies to neighborhood organizations; namely, new and still finding its way in terms of mission and goals or old and established. The history of an organization is important for understanding its present realities and future opportunities.

The stage of development continuum can be seen most vividly in the evolution of a group (e.g., a citizen's neighborhood crime watch group or an agency staff group working together to develop a funding proposal for a new service). For any group, the beginning or *forming* stage involves clarifying common interests and roles to be played (Tuchman & Jensen, 1977). The *storming* stage may involve the evolution of problem-solving processes (e.g., multiple short meetings vs. fewer long meetings). The *norming* stage usually involves the clarification and codification of some rules or guidelines for future behavior (e.g., establishing an agenda, taking minutes, voting procedures, etc.). The *performing* stage involves the allocation, implementation, and evaluation of different group-identified tasks to be completed. And finally, the *adjourning* stage can include the celebration of project completion or the designation of further work to be done by another group.

Systems of Exchange

Systems of exchange are structures designed to foster mutual support in a social environment that recognizes the central role of self-interest. In essence, if we collaborate around a particular issue, "what is in it for you" and "what is in it for me?" In this context, self-interest is a neutral term (in contrast to some of the negative connotations associated with being self-centered) that seeks to capture the nature of exchange in all human interaction (e.g., I give you money in exchange for services). Systems of exchange involve an arrangement of reciprocal giving and receiving.

When applying the concept "systems of exchange" to understanding the social environment of neighborhood communities, several dimensions emerge in relationship to community building. According to Weil (1996) community building involves the development of structures that include "activities, practices, and policies that support and foster positive connections among individuals, groups, organizations, neighborhoods, and geographic and functional communities." In essence, community building involves systems of exchange. For example, engaging members of the community to invest in the improvement of their own neighborhood includes the implicit question, "what is in it for me?" The structure might be a neighborhood advisory committee and the exchange might be the transaction of devoting time to attend/participate in meetings in exchange for a cleaner or safer neighborhood.

Systems of exchange also apply to organizations. The classic structure of exchange is the relationship between an organization and its environment. For example, state and local governments or foundations provide funding to an organization in exchange for delivering services to the community. Organizations are also sensitive to their political environments and may appoint individuals to the Board of Directors in exchange for their expertise and political connections with the larger community. Organizations are dependent upon economic, political, and social support from the larger community. As a result, organization-environment relations include important funding, policy, and communications elements that are essential in managing an organization's systems of exchange.

Groups also display multiple systems of exchange. One of the most vivid examples is found in the structure for problem-solving. For a group of board members, it might be the board meeting. For a group of staff, it might be the staff meeting or a case conference. These structures provide a venue for *exchanging* ideas and opinions within an agreed-upon system for decision-making. Essentially the system of exchange can be a problem-solving framework where participants are involved in exchanging views, sharing expertise, and identifying resources at the level of a neighborhood committee, a board committee, or a staff unit.

Diversity

The concept of diversity has come to acquire many different meanings. While understanding and responding to the diversity of clients when providing human services represents the most prevalent meaning, there are other meanings with respect to communities, groups, and organizations. When focusing on the neighborhood, diversity can be reflected in the different levels of socio-economic status reflected by the residents (e.g., a blue-collar neighborhood). Diversity can also be seen in the demography of residents who are retired, single, and young families as well as the race and ethnicity of a diverse or homogeneous neighborhood. The extent to which neighborhoods are segregated or integrated represents another aspect of communal diversity (Fellin, 2001, p. 152).

The diversity of group membership is similar to neighborhood diversity in that members may reflect diverse family, work, and religious experiences as well as differences in age, gender, race, sexual orientation. Understanding the nature of such diversity is essential for the fostering of effective group processes. For example, students in a university course may have difficulty understanding the different frames of reference being used by those asking questions or making comments unless they also have some understanding of each member's family, religious, ethnic, racial, or employment background.

And finally, diversity in human service organizations can be viewed from at least three perspectives; namely, the clients served, the staff employed, and the composition of the board of directors. The diversity of client problems or needs requires organizations to develop ways of classifying clients in order to provide them with the services that meet their needs. In contrast to client diversity, the diversity of staff can be understood, in part, by the organization's commitment to affirmative action (e.g., promoting racial and ethnic diversity) and/or staff development (e.g., promoting career advancement). Clearly the diversity of staff competence and experience affect career advancement. Other issues of diversity can be seen in the composition of the organization's board of directors with respect to the array of members reflecting different groups with respect to age, gender, race, ethnicity, and sexual orientation.

This discussion of diversity completes the description of the concepts related to structure in Figure 3. The next section focuses on the process concepts of leadership and power, conflict and change, and integration.

ELEMENTS OF PROCESS

Power and Leadership

The concepts of power and leadership are complex and can be defined in many different ways. When thinking about both concepts at the neighborhood level, the role of political and economic power come to mind. Political power may be reflected in the capacity of the neighborhood residents to promote neighborhood improvement (e.g., through the power of a local church) or lobby city hall for changes in the zoning ordinance to promote economic development and job growth in the neighborhood. In contrast, neighborhood leadership might be reflected in the cosmopolitan or local behaviors of neighborhood leaders (Warren, 1963). *Cosmopolitans* are those who have developed networks of relationships beyond the neighborhood with elected officials, business leaders, or leaders of non-profit organizations. *Locals* are those who have spent most of their time cultivating relationships and coordinating local projects with less emphasis on those outside the neighborhood. Understanding these leadership styles can help explain the use of power at the neighborhood level.

In the context of groups, power can be displayed in terms of expertise, position, and access to rewards and related networks (French & Raven, 1960). Power may be displayed through the concepts of task and process; namely the ability to help the group "stay on task" and/or use debriefing sessions to reflect on the dynamics of the group's "process." The leadership capacities of group members are essential ingredients for understanding the behaviors of a group. Those group members who utilize leadership behaviors are also able to demonstrate followership behaviors (Fiedler, 1967).

The role of power and leadership in organizations is also a complex inter-relationship. As Hasenfeld (1983) noted, human service organizations are loosely-coupled systems whereby line staff exercise considerable power in the form of discretion when providing services to clients. Similarly, managers of decentralized service programs located in satellite offices or clinics also exercise considerable power. The centralization of power in human service organizations (e.g., more tightly coupled systems) can be found in the roles played by staff in the areas of financial management and information systems. These two organizational functions reflect the use of power and control with respect to budget and information monitoring. A similar centralization of power can be found in employee unions that seek to protect employee rights and prerogatives. The leadership styles of clinicians and managers can be affected by the role of power in the operation of all aspects of human service organizations.

Conflict and Change

The concepts of conflict and change are also inter-connected. At the neighborhood level, conflicts between renter and landlords can be a source of great tension until there is a change (e.g., housing repairs, rent adjustments, etc.). Positive and negative conflicts are important components of the social environment (Coser, 1956). Positive conflict relates to issues that help bind the community together, either in opposition to an external force or as a source for engaging in a dialogue over differences (e.g., mediating property disputes). Negative conflict relates to issues that create such polarization that resolution requires considerable time and energy to resolve.

Conflict within a group takes on different characteristics from a neighborhood in that the future viability of the group can be a stake. Groups find ways to manage conflicts by implicitly or explicitly developing norms or rules to guide group processes. These norms may relate to simple issues (e.g., monitoring starting and ending times for group meetings) or complex issues related to identifying tension (e.g., interrupting group processes in order to address the tensions). As groups evolve over time, they are also changing with respect to the member's attachment to each other and/or the goals of the group. Super-ordinate goals or those goals that represent the groups reason for being are usually strong enough to provide a sufficient context for controlling or mediating conflict. For example, despite the tension among city council members in a council meeting, the group members continue to operate on a shared super-ordinate goal of representing the interests and concerns of their constituents.

Conflict and change in most organizations is a fact of life. In essence, organizations are in a constant transition from maintaining stability (frequently accompanied by a resistance to change) to fostering improvement and change (Hasenfeld, 1983). Organizations have different capacities to manage change. This capacity is often impacted by the organization's environment (e.g., financial resources and public support). Organizational resistance to change can take many forms and needs to be understood as a critical element of the organization's internal and external environment.

Integrating Mechanisms

Integrating mechanisms can be viewed as networks of relationships that hold communities, groups and organizations together or as institutionalized processes or procedures that can be used to monitor their health and well-being. In neighborhood communities, such networks include both formal and informal relationships that seek to foster the integration of the individual resident with the larger community. Tenant councils in housing complexes or neighborhood block watch groups serve as integrating mechanisms for a community. The can foster formal and informal relationships over time, as do regular meetings among the clergy whose congregations are located in the same neighborhood.

The use of integrating mechanisms in a group can be seen in the use of feedback processes or debriefing sessions at the end of each meeting in order to gather the perceptions and concerns of the members. Other integrating mechanisms include brain-storming and problem-solving processes (Patton, 2003). These processes provide a venue to surface latent group issues as well as provide structures for members to voice their concerns through a mechanism adopted by the group. In essence, the integrating mechanisms of the group provide individuals with opportunities to engage in sharing and problem-solving.

In human service organizations, integrating mechanisms can also be formal and informal. Formal staff meetings can be used to monitor ongoing agency operations in order to identify areas that need attention and problem-solving. Informal social events (celebrating birthdays and holidays) are also integrating mechanisms for fostering organizational understanding and support. Formal mechanisms like periodic accreditation can provide the organization with a set of standards by which to engage in some form of self-study. The ultimate integrating mechanism for organizations in these times of accountability and limited resources involves the measurement of performance outcomes. In this sense, organizational staff members operationalize their goals and objectives for each service program in order to gather and analyze information about clients served, community issues addressed, resources expended, and staff morale affected.

This discussion of process concepts provides a foundation, along with the previous discussion of structure concepts, for integrating both of these dimensions of the social environment when focusing on the role of the practitioner.

Practitioner-Environment Interaction

Different from the elaboration of the previous concepts related to the social environment, the interaction between practitioners and their environment represents a significantly overlooked dimension of the social environment. The focus here is on the degree to which a practitioner is able to conceptualize his or her role as an influential factor when engaging with neighbor residents, colleagues in a staff meeting, or one's supervisor or supervisees in an organizational setting. The interaction is a two-way street whereby the community, group and organization can also influence the behaviors of the practitioner. The interaction represents a key element of self-reflective practice (Schon, 1984).

In a community context, for example, a practitioner might focus on empowering the residents to engage in neighborhood organizing by articulating their concerns in order to develop their own "voice." At the same time, the community is educating the practitioner as to the local customs and traditions that have guided both formal and informal relationships. In a similar fashion, the practitioner engaged in group facilitation (formally and informally) can have a profound influence on how the group members engage with one another. At the same time, the group is educating the practitioner as to its prior experiences, use of language and/or acronyms, and patterns of formal and informal leadership within the group.

And finally, the manager as a practitioner in a human service organization can have significant influence over how staff members are treated, issues resolved, funds allocated, and information processed. At the same time, staff members can significantly influence managerial behaviors with respect to the quality of the workplace environment, the management of conflict and change, and the representation of the organization in the larger community. And finally, an understanding of the history and customs of the organization can greatly influence a practitioner's effectiveness in working with the internal and external environment of the organizations (Austin, 1996).

IMPLICATIONS AND CONCLUSION

The implications of the full framework presented above for social work practice are presented through the application of the model to the case vignette, and implications for research can be observed as a quest for normative definitions of success.

Applying the Social Environment Framework to a Case Vignette

One approach to applying the social environment framework depicted in Figure 1 is to use a case vignette. In so doing, we are drawing upon Mulroy (2004) and Mulroy and Lauber (2002) by using the issue of homelessness and the creation of a unique organization noted in Figure 2. One of the purposes of developing a comprehensive framework for understanding the social environment is to demonstrate how theoretical concepts and ideas can inform practice.

In the beginning of our analysis, we raised several questions about the societal forces at play in the case of the Housing Assistance Corporation. As was evident in the case vignette, multiple societal forces were at play in addressing homelessness. The *social justice concepts of moral sensibility and community care* are apparent in the mission of HAC to "promote and implement the right of all people to occupy safe and affordable housing." The outrage associated with low-income families living in their cars or individuals living in boxes in the local park provided the clear motivation of citizens and staff of a fledgling organization to take collective action to develop shelters and other alternatives. Out of a sense of achieving social justice, citizens and staff sought to identify the social problem of homelessness in such a way as to help locals understand that a service economy of low-wage jobs requires that attention be given to low-income housing.

Reframing the social problem issues from individual pathology to community responsibility and asset building required an understanding of the regional political economy of housing supply and demand AND the social justice consciousness to seek collective action. One approach to understanding a social problem is to search for information about how it is handled elsewhere, particularly in the form of public policy. Understanding the *nature of state and federal social policy* related to housing and income maintenance can then lead to information about how to access financial resources that are targeted to the social problem of homelessness. In addition to the presence or absence of relevant public policies, it is important to identify promising practices elsewhere in the country that seek to provide a *collective response* to the critical question: What is in the interests of all members of this community? With reframing, one can see how one set of solutions (shelters) can also confound the homeless problem by creating such dependency that individuals and families either choose to stay in shelters due to the absence of affordable housing or refuse to use shelters because they may not be safe.

As noted in the case vignette, community outreach to residents, opinion leaders, and public officials was part of a community planning initiative that involved public education and conflict mediation. The goal was to help all those impacted by the problem recognize that they were in fact stakeholders in finding solutions. Understanding the *structure* of the local community and the *processes* it uses to promote or block change was essential. While reaching out to others, HAC also needed to develop its own infrastructure (a new *stage of organizational development*) by writing/securing grants to support staff and balance its attention to shelters and to the complex process of affordable housing development. All these processes represented *systems of exchange*, learning about what needs to get done in order to secure funding. It also involved a keen understanding of the diversity of perspectives in the community as well as the socio-demographic profile of the residents, both rich and poor.

And finally, without an understanding of *group dynamics*, very little could have been accomplished. From managing public information meetings (seeking and promoting leadership among both cosmopolitans and locals) to recognizing that *change often involves conflict*, it was apparent that both staff and board members needed to know how different groups operated across the region (zoning board, economic development groups, and resistant residents with their NIMBY attorneys). The multiple levels of group dynamics relied heavily on gathering information, such as how HAC was being perceived in the community and how HAC perceived multiple sources of both support and resistance. This information provided important *integrating mechanisms* for board members and staff to maintain momentum and to equip the *leadership* with the *power* of information that helped their own group problem-solving processes.

Throughout the entire case, it was apparent that the Dana's Fields project would not have succeeded without the involvement of many people, especially one MSW program manager with an alternative vision for serving the homeless. As a practitioner in the Cape Cod environment, she recognized that she could have an impact on the social environment. This important element of *practitioner-environment interaction* provides a living example of how a comprehensive understanding of the social environment can inform practice. Effective practice requires a continuous search for relevant theoretical concepts, especially those related to the social environment, if theory is to play an ongoing role in informing practice.

Normative Definitions of Success

The delineation of the concept of the social environment raises complicated questions concerning successful outcomes. The case of the Housing Assistance Corporation is an example of local-level innovation in the nonprofit sector. The organization linked macro-systems with micro community systems to achieve basic human needs for a vulnerable population in their region–homeless individuals and families. Important research questions are raised for the future: How can a theoretical perspective be used to effectively study organizations, groups, and communities? How well do our social institutions respond to social problems? To what extent do community building endeavors as seen in the case of the Housing Assistance Corporation contribute to a healthy community? What do these issues suggest for the selection of social indicators and indices which serve as paths to understanding societal forces as trends in the lives of people?

The social work community has been concerned with the individual as the premiere unit of analysis. We suggest that this perspective does not account for the impacts and complex interplay within the social environment. The vignette of the Housing Assistance Corporation raises questions about how improved the urbanizing region had become, how effective the organization had become, and how the process of change had improved group functioning inside and outside the organization. Establishing criteria for measuring such effectiveness or improvement represents a future agenda worth pursuing. In addition, the case of the Housing Assistance Corporation and the conceptual framework of the article provide further challenges in the area of "theory for research." While current research paradigms place priority on the human behavior dimensions of the individual and family, further attention is needed in the area of social environment variables that inform the measurement of change in groups, communities, organizations, and social policies.

We consider this paper a first step in examining the initial questions set forth, and acknowledge the limitations of what we were not able to do. First, one next step would be to link the framework presented here with human behavior content. Another step would be to address the CSWE standard on the reciprocal relationship between human behavior and the social environment. Second, our attention has been on theory for practice. Work needs to be done in a similar vein to link other reciprocal relationships such as HBSE and social policy (i.e., societal forces), and HBSE and research (the ways in which theory guides, informs, and builds upon research). The long term goal is to understand the complexity of factors that comprise the social environment so that social workers can better address the perceived reciprocity between how people behave, and the conditions in the environments in which they live and work.

REFERENCES

Adams, P., & Nelson, K. (1998). *Reinventing human services: Community- and family-centered practice.* New York: Aldine DeGruyter.

Austin, M.J. (1996). Planning for organizational change: Linking the past with the present and future. *Journal of Jewish Communal Service.*

Bailey, G. (Nov. 2003). Embracing 'radical social work.' *NASW News* 48(10) 3.

Brown, L. (Ed.), (1993). *The new shorter oxford english dictionary on historical principles.* Oxford, UK: Clarendon Press.

Coser, L. (1956). *The functions of social conflict.* Glencoe, IL: Free Press.

Craig, G. (2002). Poverty, Social Work, and Social Justice. *British Journal of Social Work.* 32, 669-682.

Downs, A. (1973). *Urban Problems and Prospects.* Chicago: Markham.

Fabricant, M., & Fisher, R. (2002). *Settlement houses under siege. The struggle to sustain community organizations in New York.* New York: Columbia University Press.

Feagin, J. (1998). *The new urban paradigm: Critical perspectives on the city.* Oxford: Roman & Littlefield.

Fellin, P. (2001). *The community and the social worker.* Itasca, IL: F.E. Peacock.

Fiedler, F.E. (1967). *A theory of leadership effectiveness.* New York: McGraw Hill.

Fields, R. (Nov. 30, 2003). Losing Walker: A life of promise cut down in youth. *Baltimore Sun* p. 1.

French, J.R.P., & Raven, B. (1960). The bases of social power. *Group Dynamics,* D. Cartwright, and A. Zander (Eds.). Evanston, IL: Row, Peterson.

Frey, W. (2002). Three Americas: The rising significance of regions. *Journal of the American Planning Association.* 68(4) 349-354.

Gibelman, M., & Demone, H. Jr. (2002). The commercialization of health and human services: National phenomena or cause for concern? *Families in Society.* 83(4) 387-397.

Gil, D. (1998). *Confronting injustice and oppression.* New York: Columbia University Press.

Gottdiener, M., & Pickvance, C. (1991). Introduction. In M.Gottdiener, & C. Pickvance (Eds.), *Urban life in transition.* Vol. 39 Urban Affairs Annual Reviews. Newbury Park, CA: Sage pp. 1-11.

Gray, B. (1989). *Collaborating: Finding common ground to multiparty problems.* San Francisco: Jossey-Bass.

Hardcastle, D., Wenocur, S., & Powers, P. (1997). *Community Practice.* New York: Oxford University Press.

Harvey, D. (1973). *Social justice and the city.* Baltimore: Johns Hopkins University Press.

Hasenfeld, Y. (1983). *Human service organizations.* Upper Saddle River, NJ: Prentice-Hall.

Healey, L. (2001). *International social work.* New York: Oxford University Press.

Henry, D., Der Hovanesian, M., & Foust, D. (Nov. 10, 2003). Wall Street M & A Deals: Show Me. *Business Week* p. 38-40.

Jansson, B. (1994). *Social Policy: From theory to practice.* (2nd ed.). Pacific Grove, CA: Brooks/Cole.

Julian, J. (1977). *Social problems*. 2nd edition. Englewood Cliffs, NJ: Prentice-Hall.
Kanter, R.M. (2000). Business coalitions as a force for regionalism. In B. Katz, (Ed.), *Reflections on regionalism*. Washington, DC: The Brookings Institution. pp. 154-184.
Katz, B. (2000). Editor's overview. In B. Katz, (Ed.), *Reflections on regionalism*. Washington, DC: Brookings Institution. pp. 1-8.
Lefebrvre, H. (1991). *The production of space*. Cambridge, MA: Blackwell, Inc.
Longres, J., & Scanlon, E. (2001). Social justice and the research curriculum. *Journal of Social Work Education*. 37(3) 447-463.
Marsh, J. (2003). The Social work response to violence. Editorial. *Social Work*. 48(4) 437-438.
Meehan, E. (1979). *The quality of federal policy making: Programmed failure in public housing*. Columbia: University of Missouri Press.
Midgely, J. (2000). The definition of social policy. In J. Midgely, M. Tracy, & M. Livermore. *The handbook of social policy*. Thousand Oaks, CA: Sage. pp. 3-10.
Mier, R. & Giloth, R. (1993). Cooperative leadership for community problem solving. In R. Mier, (Ed.), *Social justice and local development policy*. Thousand Oaks, CA: Sage 165-181.
Mier, W., & Giloth, R. (1993). Spatial change and social justice. In *Social Justice and Local Development Policy*. R. Mier, (Ed.). Newbury Park, CA: Sage.
Mulroy, E. (1997). Building a neighborhood network: Interorganizational collaboration to prevent child abuse and neglect. *Social Work*. 42(3) 255-264.
Mulroy, E. (2003). Community as a factor in implementing interorganizational partnerships. *Nonprofit Management & Leadership*. 14(1) 47-66.
Mulroy, E. (2004). Theoretical perspectives on the social environment to guide management and community practice: An organization-in-environment approach. *Administration in Social Work*.
Mulroy, E., & Lauber, H. (2002). Community building in hard times: A post-welfare view from the streets. *Journal of Community Practice*. 10(1) 1-16.
Netting, F. E., Kettner, P., & McMurtry, S. (1993). *Social Work Macro Practice*. White Plains, NY: Longman.
Patton, B.R., & Downs, T.M. (2003). *Decision-making group interaction: Achieving quality*. 4th edition, Boston: Allyn & Bacon.
Rawls, J. (1971). *A theory of justice*. Cambridge, MA: Harvard University Press.
Rothman, J., Erlich, J., & Tropman, J. (2001). *Strategies of Community Intervention*. 6th edition. Itasca, IL: F.E. Peacock Publishers.
Schon, D. A. (1984). The *reflective practitioner: How professionals think in action*. NY: Basic Books.
Schorr, A. (1997). *Passion and policy*. Cleveland: David Press.
Smizik, F., & Stone, M. (1988). Single-parent families and the right to housing. In E. Mulroy, (Ed.), *Women as single parents: Confronting institutional barriers in the courts, the workplace, and the housing market*. Westport, CT: Auburn House, pp. 227-270.
Solomon, R. (1995). *A passion for justice: Emotions and the origins of the social contract*. Lanham, MD: Rowman & Littlefield.

Taylor, S., Austin, M., & Mulroy, E. (2004). Evaluating the social work component of social work courses on human behavior and the social environment. *Journal of Human Behavior in the Social Environment.* 10(3) 61-84.

Taylor, S., Mulroy, E., & Austin, M. (2004). Social work textbooks and the social environment: An analysis of the social environment component. *Journal of Human Behavior in the Social Environment.* 10(3) 85-109.

Tuchman, B.W., & M.A. Jensen (1977). Stages of small group development revisited. *Groups and Organizational Studies.* 2(1) 419-427.

Van Soest, D., & Garcia, B. (2003). *Diversity education for social justice.* Alexandria, VA: CSWE Press.

Warren, R. (1978). *The community in America.* Chicago: Rand McNally.

Weil, M. (1996). Community building: Building community practice. *Social Work.* 41(5).

Wolch, J. (1990). *The shadow state.* New York: The Foundation Center.

Wolch, J., & Dear, M. (1993). *Malign neglect: Homelessness in an American city.* San Francisco: Jossey-Bass.

Evaluating the Social Environment Component of Social Work Courses on Human Behavior and the Social Environment

Sarah Taylor
Michael J. Austin
Elizabeth A. Mulroy

SUMMARY. This analysis of 117 foundation of Human Behavior and Social Environment (HB&SE) course outlines gathered from 60 graduate schools of social work is based on the HB&SE standards of the Council on Social Work Education (2001). It draws upon an analytic framework for integrating content related to the social environment. Specific criteria for assessment included how well the course outline reflected the reciprocal nature of human behavior and the social environment, presented a strengths perspective, incorporated diversity content, and covered material related to families, groups, organizations, communities, and political economy. Four types of HB&SE course outlines were identified (*lifespan-oriented, systems-oriented, theory-oriented,* and *combination*), and results are presented by course

---

Sarah Taylor, MSW, is Doctoral Research Assistant and Michael J. Austin, PhD, (E-mail: mjaustin@berkeley.edu) is Professor, School of Social Welfare, University of California, Berkeley. Elizabeth A. Mulroy, PhD, is Associate Professor, School of Social Work, University of Maryland-Baltimore.

[Haworth co-indexing entry note]: "Evaluating the Social Environment Component of Social Work Courses on Human Behavior and the Social Environment." Taylor, Sarah, Michael J. Austin, and Elizabeth A. Mulroy. Co-published simultaneously in *Journal of Human Behavior in the Social Environment* (The Haworth Social Work Practice Press, an imprint of The Haworth Press, Inc.) Vol. 10, No. 3, 2004, pp. 61-84; and: *The Conundrum of Human Behavior in the Social Environment* (ed: Marvin D. Feit and John S. Wodarski) The Haworth Social Work Practice Press, an imprint of The Haworth Press, Inc., 2004, pp. 61-84. Single or multiple copies of this article are available for a fee from The Haworth Document Delivery Service [1-800-HAWORTH, 9:00 a.m. - 5:00 p.m. (EST). E-mail address: docdelivery@haworthpress.com].

© 2004 by The Haworth Press, Inc. All rights reserved.
Digital Object Identifier: 10.1300/J137v10n03_03

outline type. The findings suggest that increased attention to content related to the macro social environment, human diversity, well-being, and theory for practice is needed to strengthen HB&SE foundation courses.

[Article copies available for a fee from The Haworth Document Delivery Service: 1-800-HAWORTH. E-mail address: <docdelivery@ haworthpress.com> Website: <http://www. HaworthPress.com> © 2004 by The Haworth Press, Inc. All rights reserved.]

KEYWORDS. Social environment, social environment in HB&SE courses

INTRODUCTION

The variation in Human Behavior and Social Environment (HB&SE) courses in Social Work programs reflects the continuing debates about how social and behavioral science theories should inform social work practice (Brooks, 1986; Farley, Smith, Boyle, & Ronnau, 2002; Mailick & Vigilante, 1987). The debate focuses primary attention either on the behavior of individuals or on the impact of the social environment on the behavior of individuals and families. Since the "rise and fall" of the psychoanalytic perspective (Mohan, 1980, p. 26), social work educators have searched for ways to include more content on the social environment as well as alternative theoretical constructs, especially as they seek to balance the concepts of pathology with those of well-being. One of the results of this searching process, according to Levande (1987, p. 59), has been an "add and stir" method that involves introducing new content into an increasingly packed agenda that " . . . can result in HBSE content that is contradictory [and] fragmented . . . "

HB&SE is a core component of the foundation of a social work curriculum. It competes for curricular "shelf space" with social work practice, social policy, social research, field work, and content related to values and ethics, human diversity, populations-at-risk, and social justice (Council on Social Work Education, 2001). As a core component, one way to assess HB&SE content is to review the way courses and most frequently cited textbooks are structured. This assessment focuses heavily on the social environment content in HB&SE courses and is part of a larger study that includes the development of a comprehensive conceptual framework of the social environment (Mulroy & Austin, 2004) and a review of HB&SE textbooks (Taylor, Mulroy, & Austin, 2004). This study features a review of 117 HB&SE course outlines gathered from 60 accredited graduate schools of social work.

The focal point for this analysis was the most current CSWE (2001) curriculum statement on HB&SE content as cited below (italics added): Social work education programs provide content on the *reciprocal relationships between human behavior and social environments*. Content includes empirically based theories and knowledge that focus on the interactions between and among individuals, groups, societies, and economic systems. It includes theories and knowledge of biological, sociological, cultural, psychological, and spiritual development across the *life span*; the range of *social systems* in which people live (individual, family, group, organizational, and community); and the ways social systems promote or deter people in maintaining or achieving health and *well-being* (Council on Social Work Education, 2001, p. 35).

LITERATURE REVIEW

In searching the literature as far back as the 1960s, we found only two empirical studies on the content and organization of HB&SE courses (Brooks, 1986; Farley et al., 2002). The lack of research on HB&SE is surprising given its centrality within the social work curriculum.

The majority of the HB&SE literature consists of scholarly essays on the controversies related to teaching HB&SE. Mailick and Vigilante (1987) identified the following five major controversies in teaching HB&SE: (1) the over-emphasis on psychoanalytic theories; (2) the limitations of organizing content by developmental stages; (3) the need for more content on social stress and coping; (4) the call for more human diversity content; and (5) the difficulty in differentiating between BSW and MSW level HB&SE course content.

To address these HB&SE curricular issues, social work educators have proposed several conceptual frameworks. Hunter and Saleebey (1977) suggest that HB&SE should balance "a superordinate ideal of freedom and a central, integrating idea or theory of alienation" (p. 60). The freedom concept refers to promoting social justice and the theory of alienation provides the analytic foundation for engaging in social action.

Others have advocated for the application of Vance's (1973) theory of "social disability" to the teaching of HB&SE (Schlesinger & Schatz, 1977). Social ability is conceptualized as a continuum ranging from socially disabled to socially competent. Social competence is influenced by human interaction with the environment, which consists of the following dimensions: ". . . moderateness, orderliness (pattern), rhythmicity, density (of population), responsiveness, threatfulness, an over or understimulating dimension, consistency-inconsistency of reinforcement, power-powerlessness" (p. 85). The authors suggest that social disability is a useful lens for analyzing poverty and other social problems in HB&SE courses.

Mailick and Vigilante (1987) emphasize the application of theory to practice. They envision HB&SE courses organized around a "developmental wheel" (p. 41) that includes four rings: The outermost ring symbolizes "basic human aspirations" such as protection and social justice; the next ring represents intervening variables such as role, family, and culture; the second ring includes social pathologies such as classism, racism, and sexism; and the innermost ring relates to individual human developmental needs.

Levande (1987) suggests that HB&SE courses should include the following seven elements: (1) social work as a profession; (2) systems theory and the ecological perspective; (3) interaction theories within a systems perspective; (4) biological perspectives; (5) the meso environment; (6) the macro environment; and (7) theories of individual human behavior. Others argue for the inclusion of more content on social work policy (Mohan, 1980), as well as an emphasis on learning about theories and acquiring critical thinking skills (Guidry, 1979; Miller, 1981).

The diversity of these perspectives is captured in the limited amount of research based on HB&SE course descriptions (Brooks, 1986) and course outlines (Farley et al., 2002). Brooks (1986) analyzed 481 graduate HB&SE course descriptions printed in course catalogs from 66 schools of social work. The analysis focused on three key questions: (1) Was the course identifiable as having a macro or micro focus? (While "micro" and "macro" are not specifically defined, they correspond roughly to human behavior and the social environment, respectively); (2) Did micro courses cover more than one theory?; and (3) Did course descriptions note the incorporation of human diversity content? Of the 481 courses analyzed, 300 (62%) were identified as having either a macro or micro focus, a finding that the author suggests indicates a separation, rather than integration, of HB&SE content. The remaining 38% of courses were specialty courses addressing specific social problems or populations. Another major finding was that 78% of the 300 courses that could be identified as either micro or macro, focused on individual human behavior. Additionally, only 11% of the courses specified that the course incorporated diversity content.

Farley et al. (2002) evaluated 116 HB&SE course outlines used in 61 MSW programs during the 1998-1999 academic year. The authors present findings in five categories: (1) sequencing of courses; (2) theoretical constructs; (3) course objectives; (4) course requirements; and (5) textbooks and readings. They found that 72% of the schools offered two foundation HB&SE courses and 20% offered one, with the remaining schools offering three or more. Of those schools offering two HB&SE courses, 52% devoted one semester to life cycle, and the other to the social environment as represented by content on groups, organizations, and communities. Another 21% of the schools focused on life cycle in the first semester and other topics the second semester, including human diversity, oppression, and systems perspectives. Several schools (17%) offering two HB&SE courses over two semesters that either taught the life cycle in both semesters or focused on normal development one semester and abnormal development in the second semester. Only 20% of course outlines had a focus on social justice, populations-at-risk, discrimination, or culture. Because of the wide variation in HB&SE course outlines, Farley et al. (2002) concluded that HB&SE courses continue to reflect a lack of agreement about core content and theoretical constructs. They also noted that the courses needed to increase coverage of human diversity issues and populations-at-risk.

When comparing the Brooks (1986) study with the Farley et al. study (2002), published sixteen years later, some interesting findings emerge. Brooks (1986) found that 62% of the course descriptions had either a micro or macro focus, and similarly, Farley et al. (2002) found that 52% of the schools offered two HB&SE courses where one semester was devoted to human behavior and the other to the social environment. This suggests that between 1986 and 1998 (the year of the course outlines analyzed by Farley et al.), the majority of HB&SE courses reflected a continuing bifurcation between content on human behavior and social environments. While Brooks (1986) noted that only 11% of course descriptions incorporated human diversity content, Farley et al. (2002) found that human diversity content had increased to 20%.

Our analysis builds on the work of Brooks (1986) and Farley et al. (2002) by examining HB&SE course outlines of MSW programs from the 2002-2003 academic year, and focuses on the following key research questions:

1. How well do course outlines adhere to the CSWE (2001) guidelines for HB&SE curriculum, including specification and *integration* of material on human behavior and the social environment?

2. How are courses organized (by units on systems, theories, stages of the lifespan, or other) and how well do these different course types meet the CSWE (2001) guidelines?
3. How well do HB&SE course outlines demonstrate the integration of human diversity content?

Given the revised CSWE guidelines on HB&SE curriculum (2001), and the challenge of incorporating human diversity content, it seems timely to re-evaluate HB&SE courses by using the most current data available.

METHODS

An e-mail request was sent to the deans of 156 accredited MSW programs in the Spring of 2003 based on the most current directory (Council on Social Work Education, 2002). The specific request called for sending a copy of course outlines for all *the required foundation HB&SE courses* offered by their MSW program (not advanced HB&SE electives). A total of 60 schools responded (a 38% response rate) by sending 117 course outlines. The participating schools were fairly representative of social work schools nationally in terms of region, school size, reputation, and curricular emphases (i.e., research, clinical social work, social justice). The first step in the analysis involved the identification of basic demographics (e.g., total number of outlines and number of schools offering one, two, or three or more HB&SE courses, etc.). Five syllabi were then selected at random and reviewed thoroughly to identify variability in the sample and to develop a set of criteria (based on the research questions) for use in assessing each course outline.

Based on the review of the five outlines, it became clear that the typology (*theory*, *systems*, and *lifespan* types) that emerged from our study of HB&SE textbooks (Taylor et al., 2004) would be useful in the analysis of course outlines as well.

Theory-oriented courses are those that focus predominantly on the specification of various theoretical perspectives, such as systems theory, psychodynamic theory, and cognitive behavioral theory.

Systems-oriented courses are structured around social system elements (individuals, families, small groups, organizations, communities, and societies). Individuals are often described as being one type or size of system, and all systems are described as interdependent entities irrespective of how individuals experience them.

Lifespan-oriented courses include the specification of various stages of human development from infancy through old age. Some of these course outlines also include sections on various systems (groups, organizations, and communities), but the majority of the content emphasizes the life cycle.

A course outline was classified into one of these three categories if more than 50% of the course outline reflected one of these types. As outlines were classified, two other types emerged. Several outlines were classified as "combination" outlines in which material seemed evenly divided between lifespan, theory, and/or systems. A small number of outlines were classified as "specialized" and focused primarily on psychopathology or diversity.

Based on the CSWE accreditation guidelines on HB&SE curriculum content and a careful review of the five randomly selected outlines, eight criteria were developed for evaluating each course outline and are described in Figure 1. The first four relate to the CSWE guidelines, while the remaining four emerged from our study of the randomly selected outlines.

Outlines were then reviewed individually. A tally sheet was completed for each group of outlines (systems, theory, lifespan, and combination). Results are not reported for course outlines classified as "specialized" (n = 18) since these courses appeared to be too specific in focus (examples of primary topics included psychopathology, history of oppression, and international human rights). A final step in the analysis process included selecting and summarizing four prototype outlines, one from each group, to show how outlines met our criteria.

There are several limitations to this study. While there was an extensive search of the literature for similar analyses of HB&SE courses, only two studies could be found even though others may exist. Second, there were insufficient financial and human resources to develop a comprehensive, in-depth assessment of each outline. Third, the outlines were evaluated by only two of the three co-authors. And fourth, course outlines are an imperfect measure for assessing the content or the delivery of the course content. Future studies should include instructor surveys or interviews, as well as observations of how course content is being presented.

FINDINGS

The findings are presented in three sections and noted in Table 1. The first section includes the overall demographics of the sample and the

FIGURE 1. Eight Criteria for Assessing HB&SE Course Outlines

Description of Criteria	Location in Course Outline
1. Reciprocal relationship between HB&SE–defined as the dynamic, interdependent nature of the relationship between human behavior and social environments, reflecting a unified, complex whole, whereby human behavior and social environments influence one another, (rather than a one-way relationship in which human behavior is shaped by the social environment).	Explicitly stated in the course description and/or objectives
2. Lifespan–defined as including content on human development over the lifespan.	
3. Systems–defined as including content on systems of varying sizes, including families, groups, organizations, and communities.	
4. Well-being–defined as emphasizing as strengths, well-being, wellness, or adaptive functioning perspective.	
5. Comparative perspectives–defined as the presentation of multiple perspectives for understanding human behavior and social environments, and the critical evaluation of alternative perspectives.	
6. Logical flow–defined as logical and coherent sequencing of course content (not the "add and stir" approach described by Levande (1987)).	Revealed through a review of entire course outline
7. Incorporation of diversity content–defined as the integration of human diversity content (not relegated to one or two class sessions) as indicated by either required readings throughout the course or detailed descriptions of diversity topics in more than two class sessions.	
8. Theory for practice–defined as at least one course assignment designed to apply HB&SE concepts to practice situations (e.g., constructing a genogram, analyzing a case from multiple theoretical perspectives, applying concepts to one's own stage of development).	Reflected in descriptions of course assignments

number of foundation HB&SE courses offered. The second section includes findings related to the eight assessment criteria for evaluating HB&SE courses. The final section provides highlights of four prototypic course outlines (systems, theory, mix, and lifespan).

Types of HB&SE Courses Offered

The findings are based on an analysis of 117 course outlines sent by 60 schools of social work with accredited MSW programs. Of the 60 schools, we found that 58% (35) offer two foundation HB&SE courses, while 33% (20) offer one, and the remaining 8% schools (5) offer three or more.

Overall, the findings reflect a diverse array of approaches to structuring HB&SE content. Of the 35 schools offering two HB&SE courses, 31% (11) devoted one semester to lifespan, and the second semester to

TABLE 1. Application of Eight Criteria to Four Types of Course Outlines

Types of Course Outlines	1. CSWE Reciprocal Relationship between HB&SE	2. CSWE Lifespan	3. CSWE Systems	4. CSWE Wellbeing	Total of CSWE-based criteria	5. Comparative Perspectives	6. Logical Flow	7. Incorporation of Diversity Content	8. Theory for Practice
1. Systems n = 23	73% (16/22)	55% (12/22)	100% (22/22)	55% (12/22)	70% (62/88)	59% (13/22)	91% (21/23)	80% (16/20)	100% (14/14)
2. Theory n = 16	44% (7/16)	56% (9/16)	69% (11/16)	56% (9/16)	56% (36/64)	75% (12/16)	81% (13/16)	33% (5/15)	56% (5/9)
3. Lifespan n = 33	75% (24/32)	100% (32/32)	63% (20/32)	38% (12/32)	69% (88/128)	63% (20/32)	100% (33/33)	79% (15/19)	58% (15/26)
4. Combination n = 27	41% (11/27)	52% (14/27)	52% (14/27)	52% (14/27)	49% (53/108)	78% (21/27)	48% (13/27)	65% (15/23)	55% (11/20)
Percent of all outlines	60% (58/97)	69% (67/97)	69% (67/97)	48% (47/97)	62% (239/388)	68% (66/97)	81% (80/99)	66% (51/77)	65% (45/69)

systems, while 17% (6) presented a combination of lifespan, systems, and theory material over two semesters. Another 11% (4) schools covered lifespan in the first semester, and did a combination of theory, systems, and diversity in the second semester. Three schools (9%) focused on systems during the first semester, and theory in the second semester. One school presented the lifespan over two semesters, while another school presented systems over two semesters. The remaining 3% (9) taught systems, theory, or lifespan in one semester, and diversity, psychopathology, or a combination of topics in the other.

Of the 20 schools requiring only one foundation HB&SE course (several schools sent different versions of the same course outline, thus proportions given are based on the outlines received), 35% (9) focused on the lifespan, 19% (5) emphasized systems, and another 19% (5) presented primarily theories. The remaining outlines (8) reflected a combination of theory, diversity, lifespan, and systems.

The three schools that required three foundation HB&SE courses and the two schools that required four foundation HB&SE courses also varied in the content and structure of their courses. The multiple components of these courses can be described as follows: (1) theory, direct practice, systems; (2) combination lifespan and psychopathology, theory, combination theory and systems; (3) theory, combination diversity and social problems, lifespan; (4) community practice, organizational practice, individual practice, assessment; (5) combination theory and lifespan, lifespan, psychopathology, diversity. Given the mix of content, it is not clear where HB&SE ends and practice content begins.

Application of the Eight Criteria

Table 1 summarizes the extent to which the course outlines reflected the eight criteria defined in Figure 1. The results are reported in a format that uses the four main types of courses: systems (n = 23), lifespan (n = 33), theory (n = 16), or combination (n = 27).

In the process of evaluating outlines, those that did not provide sufficient information for assessing a particular criterion were excluded from the final percentages. For example, several outlines did not give any information about assignments; therefore, the percentage of outlines that met our "theory for practice" criterion is based *only* on those outlines that provided sufficient information.

CSWE HB&SE Standards

A substantial majority of both systems-oriented (70%) and lifespan-oriented (69%) HB&SE course outlines successfully incorporated the CSWE (2001) guidelines based on the four assessment criteria (e.g., reciprocal relationship between HB&SE, lifespan, systems, and well-being). This compares to 56% of the theory-oriented outlines and 49% of the combination outlines. With respect to the lifespan outlines, 75% describe the relationship between human behavior and the social environment as reciprocal. Most of the systems outlines (73%) also noted the reciprocal nature of HB&SE. Less than half of the combination outlines (41%) and theory outlines (44%) described human behavior and the social environment as interdependent perspectives. Of the 97 outlines evaluated, 48% reflected a wellness or strengths perspective in the course description or objectives.

Comparative Perspectives: A substantial majority of both theory (75%) and combination (78%) outlines noted in the course objectives or course description that students would learn to compare critically and/or evaluate multiple theoretical perspectives. A slightly smaller percentage of lifespan (63%) and systems (59%) outlines emphasized comparative perspectives.

Logical Flow: It was not surprising to find that all lifespan outlines demonstrated a logical flow given the nature of the sequencing of the content from birth to death. A high percentage of theory (81%) and systems (91%) outlines also flowed logically as compared to the combination outlines, where less than half (48%) appeared to present material in a logical or coherent manner that was evident from reading the course outline.

Integration of Diversity Content: An average of two-thirds of all outlines (in which adequate information was provided) reflected an integration of diversity content into either weekly topics or required readings. However, course outlines varied widely. Systems (80%) and lifespan (79%) outlines incorporated diversity content more consistently than combination (65%) and theory (33%) outlines.

Theory for Practice: All of the systems outlines that provided adequate information about assignments had at least one assignment emphasizing theory for practice. This compares to approximately half of the theory (56%), lifespan (58%), and combination (55%) outlines.

Prototype Course Outlines

Summaries of four prototype course outlines are noted in Appendices 1-4 (Montgomery, 2001; Perez Foster, 2002; Stone, 2002; Vanderbeek, 2002). Emphasis is added by using italics. Whenever possible, prototypes were selected on the basis of meeting all eight criteria for analysis as noted in Figure 1. While none of the systems or theory outlines met all eight of the criteria due to insufficient information (e.g., lack of detail on readings or assignments), the systems-oriented outline (Vanderbeek, 2002) and the theory-oriented outline (Montgomery, 2001) met at least seven criteria. Each of the four prototype course outlines incorporated the CSWE, HB&SE standards in different ways.

Discussion

When comparing the findings in this analysis with the Brooks (1986) and Farley et al. study (2002), some interesting themes emerge, particularly in the areas of integrating content on diversity and well-being.

There appears to be an increase in attention given to integrating diversity content into HB&SE courses. In our analysis, 66% of the outlines indicated that required readings and/or weekly topics throughout the semester relate HB&SE concepts to human diversity issues. In contrast, Brooks (1986) found that 11% of course descriptions incorporated diversity content, and Farley et al. (2002) found that only 20% of outlines reflected a focus on populations-at-risk, social justice, discrimination, or culture. While this increase appears promising, our data also indicate that one-third of HB&SE courses did not reflect much attention to human diversity issues.

An additional comparison with previous studies relates to well-being versus pathology. Brooks (1986) found that 32.5% of micro HB&SE courses focused primarily on psychoanalysis or psychopathology, while Farley et al. (2002) note that the course outlines reflected an overall shift away from the psychopathology focus of the 1960s and 1970s. We found that, in 2002-2003, 48% of the outlines emphasized well-being in the course objectives. While there may be a shift away from the psychopathology focus, it is not clear that a complementary shift towards well-being has taken place. This may be complicated by the increase in human diversity content and the complexity of problems facing populations-at-risk. Future research is needed to identify the best way to balance the teaching of a well-being perspective while attending to an increased understanding of social problems and oppression experienced by populations-at-risk.

Towards a Framework for Building the SE Component of HB&SE

As described in the introduction, a special focus of our analysis of HB&SE outlines is the incorporation of SE concepts into the HB&SE curriculum, and the literature review indicated that HB&SE content typically emphasizes HB at the expense of "shelf space" for SE. Perhaps one reason for this imbalance in the curriculum stems from avoidance of the "add and stir" approach in which material is fragmented (Levande, 1987).

Mulroy and Austin (2004) present a framework for selecting and organizing course content (see Figure 2) that seeks to define social environment content for integrating material into HB&SE courses. Their framework suggests that four primary forces of the macro social environment (social justice, political economy, social problems, and social policy) influence the micro social environments of communities, organizations, and groups. In their framework, the impact of the macro social environment is mediated by collective responses or collaborative efforts to address these forces. Figure 2 illustrates that as the horizontal and vertical linkages between these entities are constantly in flux, and as the societal forces change, the landscape of the social environment shifts. The framework seeks to promote an understanding of the complex macro social environment, in which globalization, privatization, immigration, and other major social forces shape the constellation of

FIGURE 2. Macro Perspective of the Social Environment: Influences of Societal Level Macro-Systems Forces on Local Micro-Systems Conditions and Dynamics

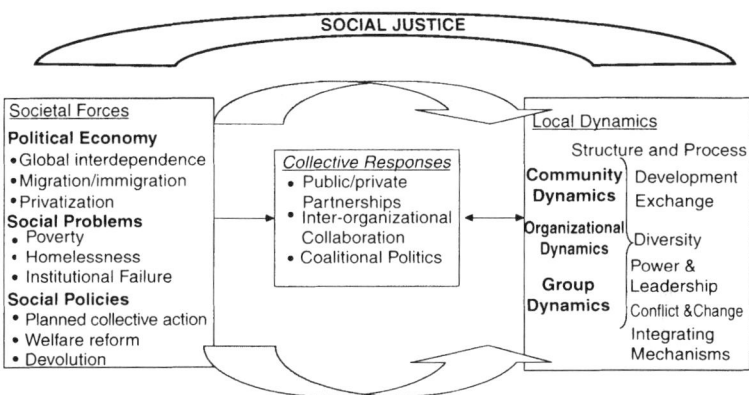

social, political, and economic relations in small towns, major metropolitan areas, and nations alike.

We applied the Mulroy and Austin (2004) framework to the twenty-three systems-oriented outlines described earlier. Though many lifespan and theory outlines include material on the social environment, we applied the framework primarily to one or more of the criteria noted in Figure 3. For some raters, the specification of the criteria in the course description or homework assignment was sufficient. For others, it needed to be noted in the outline of weekly sessions to be considered as truly reflected in the course outline.

While almost all systems-oriented HB&SE courses addressed content related to the micro system concepts of groups, organizations, and communities, only one course outline received positive scores from all three raters for also including considerable coverage of macro systems concepts related to social justice, political economy, social problems, social policies, and collective responses. As noted in Appendix 5, the application of the Mulroy and Austin (2004) framework concepts is described in relationship to this prototype systems-oriented HB&SE outline (Reed, 2002).

FIGURE 3. Mulroy and Austin (2004) Social Environment Framework Criteria

Social Justice–Redistribution of rights, resources, and power and amelioration of structural inequalities.		
Political Economy–Exploration of the complex, interdependent relationship between politics and economy in communities and larger societies, including the impact of globalization.		
Social Problems–Macro-level problems that are documented objectively through facts that attest to their persistence and/or growth over time. There must also be a perception shared by many people that these problems should be addressed.		
Social Policies–A formally organized collective response to a social problem, usually developed and managed by governmental bodies and/or agencies.		
Collective Responses–Non-governmental and/or less formally organized collaborative efforts to address the effects of social problems and policies and seek solutions toward social change.		
Structure–Includes the components of these systems and their relationships to one another within the system.	**Communities**–i.e., the specific constellation of merchants, schools, public services, etc.	
	Organizations–i.e., size, distribution of employees and work	
	Groups–i.e., membership and leadership	
Process–Includes the interactions of these components as they work towards their objectives.	**Communities**–i.e., type and degree of collaboration between entities	
	Organizations–i.e., type of relations between line staff and management	
	Groups–i.e., selection of leaders and members	

IMPLICATIONS AND CONCLUSIONS

As with most applied research, caution is needed in interpreting our findings given that only 38% of the schools of social work responded to the call for copies of course outlines. However, we think the response is adequate for an exploratory study but not sufficient for a definitive study.

One of the key findings of this study echoes Farley et al. (2002) that HB&SE courses continue to reflect a lack of agreement about core content and theoretical constructs. This is interesting given the fact that when Farley et al. collected their data, the CSWE (2001) guidelines for HB&SE had not yet been issued but were available to all schools in our study. It is possible that the CSWE guidelines are sufficiently broad as to allow for considerable variations in the development of HB&SE course content.

It was helpful to learn that 58% of the responding schools have at least two foundation HB&SE courses; however, it is not clear if this percentage is high, low, or about the same for all 154 MSW programs. It is clear from this response that a sizeable number of programs have decided that the volume of HB&SE content requires at least two courses for adequate coverage.

When it comes to the CSWE standards and the criteria for HB&SE curricula, it was interesting to note that most of the courses that featured either a life-span approach or a systems approach met most of the criteria. These included: (a) positing the reciprocal relationship between human behavior and the social environment, (b) reflecting the lifespan, (c) including systems concepts related to family, groups, organizations, and communities, and (d) focusing on well-being and the adaptive nature of the strengths perspective. However, given the brevity of the course outlines, it was not always clear how the instructor envisioned the reciprocal relationship between HB and SE, namely, how does one impact, enhance, or interfere with the other? Similarly, when courses reflecting either systems or lifespan perspectives referred to fostering comparative analyses, it was not always clear how this was carried out in lectures, readings or assignments. With regard to other CSWE standards, there is good news to report that increasing attention is being given to diversity in most HB&SE foundation courses with the exception of those courses that focus on theory. This is somewhat surprising, given the prominence of acculturation theories as well as the growing attention in the literature to the balance between a pathology and wellness orientation in understanding human behavior.

Since HB&SE courses are viewed as both an integration of the relevant bio-psycho-social sciences and a foundation for creating a synthesis of understanding designed to inform the *assessment* of human behavior and the social environment, our efforts to identify "theory for practice" produced mixed results. Our operating assumption that a student's synthesis and application of theory for practice could be most readily found in the course assignments was only partially confirmed. While many of the assignments were either related to self-assessment or case application, it was not clear how students were being assisted in linking their understanding of HB&SE to interventions at the level of the individual, group, organization, and community. This issue might be addressed more clearly if the HB&SE course outlines made more explicit the relationship between understanding human behavior and social environment concepts and the use of these concepts in formulating practice-based assessments (e.g., using the lifespan perspective related to child development and child welfare services, family dynamics and family services, adult development and health/mental health services, gerontology and aging services).

In addition to the overall assessment of HB&SE courses, our other focus was to identify the social environment content in foundation HB&SE courses. In particular, the CSWE call for elaborating the reciprocal relationship between human behavior and the social environment is predicated on the explication of both content areas as well and the dynamics between them. We began by using the explication of the social environment content found in the most frequently used HB&SE textbooks and further analytic work by Mulroy and Austin (2004). As was noted, those MSW programs with only one foundation HB&SE course focused most of their attention on human behavior with very little attention to the social environment. In those programs with two HB&SE courses, they appeared to be quite separate courses (frequently taught by different instructors) with very little apparent connection between the two courses with the exception of some share course objectives. There appeared to be no specification of cross- cutting concepts that would inform the reciprocal relationship human behavior and the social environment. Similarly, there was little evidence of course connection or integration between the HB&SE courses and the other foundation courses related to generalist social work practice or social policy.

As noted earlier, we only found one course outline that reflected a comprehensive view of the social environment (major social forces, collective responses, and major local forces related to groups, organizations, and communities). Until more attention is given to explicating the nature of the social environment, its relationship to human behavior, and its relationship to informing practice, the status quo can be expected to continue. Several questions for future research seem worth pursuing: (1) What is the reciprocal relationship between human behavior and the social environment and how is it taught? (2) What is the relationship between the backgrounds of the HB&SE instructors and the teaching of HB&SE (e.g., are predominantly psychologically-oriented clinical faculty teaching HB and sociologically-oriented macro-practice faculty (if any) teaching SE)? (3) What is really meant by "theory for practice" and how is this manifest in curriculum integration between HB&SE and practice and policy courses? and finally, (4) To what extent have social work faculty relied too heavily on our textbook authors to do the "heavy lifting" with respect to synthesizing the bio-psycho-social sciences and thereby produced brief course outlines that rely primarily on the content in the textbooks? It is a matter of speculation as to where and when these questions might be addressed in the years ahead.

In conclusion, until the social environment content of HB&SE receives the same level of attention, teaching expertise, and textbook integration as the human behavior content has received over the past decades, it can be seen as peripheral to the understanding of social work practice. The consequences of this condition could be substantial if future practitioners are not assisted in understanding the role of the social environment in the lives of clients, the daily work of agency personnel, the survival and relevance of agencies, and the community's understanding of client services.

REFERENCES

Brooks, W. (1986). Human behavior/social environment: Past and present, future or folly? *Journal of Social Work Education, 22*(1), 18-23.

Council on Social Work Education. (2001). *Handbook of Accreditation Standards and Procedures*. Alexandria, VA.

Council on Social Work Education. (2002). *Directory of College and Universities with Accredited Social Work Degree Programs*. Alexandra, VA.

Farley, O., Smith, L., Boyle, S., & Ronnau, J. (2002). A review of foundation MSW human behavior courses. *Journal of Human Behavior in the Social Environment, 6*(2), 1-12.

Guidry, R. (1979). A design for teaching human behavior in a generalist undergraduate program. *Journal of Education for Social Work, 15*(2), 45-50.

Hunter, M., & Saleebey, D. (1977). Spirit and substance: Beginnings in the education of radical social workers. *Journal of Education for Social Work, 13*(2), 60-67.

Levande, D. (1987). Boundary issues and transformation possibilities in the HBSE curriculum. *Journal of Social Work Education, 23*(3), 59-66.

Mailick, M., & Vigilante, F. (1987). Human behavior and the social environment: A sequence providing the theoretical base for teaching assessment. *Journal of Teaching in Social Work, 1*(2), 33-47.

Miller, D. (1981). Service delivery models for social work practice: Organizing the content of human behavior and social environment courses. *Journal of Education for Social Work, 17*(1), 88-95.

Mohan, B. (1980). Human behavior, social environment, social reconstruction, and social policy: A system of linkages, goals, and priorities. *Journal of Education for Social Work, 16*(2), 26-32.

Montgomery, M. (2001). Theoretical Bases of Human Behavior. California State University, Sacramento.

Mulroy, E., & Austin, M. (2004). *Towards a comprehensive framework for understanding the social environment: In search of theory for practice*. Unpublished manuscript, Baltimore, MD.

Perez Foster, R. (2002). Human Behavior in the Social Environment I: Master Outline. New York University.

Reed, B. (2002). SW 502: Organizational, Community, and Societal Structures and Processes. University of Michigan School of Social Work.

Schlesinger, E., & Schatz, J. (1977). Competence and social disability: A conceptual framework for HBSE content. *Journal of Education for Social Work, 13*(3), 84-90.

Stone, S. (2002). Human Behavior and the Social Environment. University of California, Berkeley.

Taylor, S., Mulroy, E., & Austin, M. (2004). *Social work textbooks on human behavior and the social environment: An analysis of the social environment component.* Unpublished manuscript, Berkeley, CA.

Vanderbeek, B. (2002). Human Behavior and the Social Environment. University of Iowa.

APPENDIX 1. Combination HB&SE Course Outline (Perez Foster, 2002)

Criteria	How Met	
Reciprocal Relationships	Described in first course objective: "To *conceptualize relationships among* the individual, family, group, community, environment and organizations, and *understand how these systems interact* to provide the context for human development from birth, through later childhood." This idea is reiterated in the course description: "... [the course] stresses a non-linear view of development in which there is *continuous reciprocal interchange and mutual impact among different systems (individual, family, group, community)."*	
Lifespan	Described in first course objective: "To conceptualize relationships among the individual, family, group, community, environment and organizations, and understand how these systems interact to provide the *context for human development from birth, through later childhood."*	
Systems	Described in first course objective: "To conceptualize relationships among the *individual, family, group, community, environment and organizations, and understand how these systems* interact to provide the context for human development from birth, through later childhood."	
Well-Being	Described in course objective #7: "To define the stressors and risks that may effect people from birth through late childhood; *as well as the compensatory interactions of personal, familial, group, and organizational factors that can mitigate against the negative developmental impact of these factors."*	
Comparative Perspectives	Outlined in the course description: "The course stresses the need for *the development of critical thinking throughout, an examination of the gaps in knowledge* that exists in developmental theory..."	
Logical Flow	The course begins by introducing the systems and biopsychosocial approaches, and presents separate units on biological, psychological, and social theories and concepts that contribute to the understanding of human development. The social environment concepts include family, organization, and community. The remaining three sessions of the course describe infant and child development while integrating all of the preceding material.	
Diversity	Required readings for over 1/2 the classes relate concepts to human differences in race, ethnicity, culture, gender, sexual orientation, and/or class.	
Theory for Practice	Students are asked to apply a biopsychosocial and/or systems perspective to the analysis of characters in novels and short stories	
Outline of Weekly Topics	1. The system perspective and biopsychosocial approach 2. Race, culture, and diversity 3. community and organizational systems 4. Family life in the urban environment 5. Environmental stressors and social hazzards 6. Biological/physical factors in early human development 7. Value assumptions in developmental theory	8. Cognitive development 9. Theories of attachment 10. Psychosocial theories 11. Psychoanalytic theories 12. Behaviorism and social learning theory 13. Perinatal, infant, and early childhood (applications of theories to life stage) 14. Middle and late childhood 15. Loss and bereavement in children's lives

APPENDIX 2. Lifespan-Oriented HB&SE Course (Stone, 2002)

Criteria	How Met
Reciprocal Relationships	Outlined in the course description: "This course examines *the nature of interaction*, from a developmental perspective, *between individuals and larger social systems* (with a specific focus on families, communities, and larger socio-political-cultural institutions)."
Lifespan	Outlined in the course description: "Finally, this course outlines the bio-psycho-social aspects of *major developmental stages (early childhood, middle childhood, adolescence, early and middle adulthood, and later adulthood)."*
Systems	Outlined in the course description: "This course examines the nature of interaction, from a developmental perspective, between individuals and *larger social systems* (with a specific focus on families, communities, and larger socio-political-cultural institutions)."
Well-Being	Outlined in the course description: *"It is important to note that many developmental texts are written from the perspective of individual processes (versus a person-in-environment perspective), many are written from the perspective of psychopathology (versus health), and many lack attention to human diversity."*
Comparative Perspectives	Outlined in the course description: *"This course will place a special emphasis on critiquing these theories/models* in terms of (1) existing empirical support and (2) their utility in accounting for the variability of human experience."
Logical Flow	The first four classes present background on traditional and alternative perspectives on human development and provide content on a generalist framework for social work. The remaining classes follow the life course chronologically.
Diversity	Almost all classes include required reading that relate concepts to human differences in race, ethnicity, culture, gender, sexual orientation, and/or class.
Theory for Practice	Students are asked to develop an intervention for a client, population, or social issue based on application of theoretical concepts studied in and out of the classroom
Outline of Weekly Topics	1. Overview of the course 2. Traditional formulations [of development] and critiques 3. Building a generalist framework 4. Conceptualizing the life course 5. Infancy and early childhood: Background 6. Infancy and early childhood: Context 7. School-aged children: Background 8. School-aged children: Context 9. Adolescence and youth: Background 10. Adolescence and youth: Context 11. Early to Mid Adulthood: Background 12. Early to Mid Adulthood: Context 13. Mid to Later Life: Background 14. Mid to Later Life: Context 15. Course wrap-up

APPENDIX 3. Theory-Oriented HB&SE Outline (Montgomery, 2001)

Criteria	How Met
Reciprocal Relationships	Described in course objectives: "The HBSE sequence of courses shall consider and promote student understanding of **the dynamic interaction between biological, cultural, psychological, and social systems affecting human capacity, resilience, risk, strength, and vulnerability.**" (Boldface in original.)
Lifespan	Outlined in course description: "The Fall Semester course (SW 235A) *examines human growth and development from conception/prenatal through death and dying* in the context of family, community, and society."
Systems	Outlined in course description: "The Fall Semester course (SW 235A) examines **human growth and development** from conception/prenatal through death and dying **in the context of family, community, and society.**" Course objectives 1 & 2 reiterate this by stating that student will learn and learn to apply theoretical frameworks "... **across various human systems including the family and small group, organization, community, and societal systems.**" (Boldface in original.)
Well-Being	Outlined in the course description: "The course perspective is strongly **centered in client strengths and discerning client resilience within oppressive environments.**" This is reiterated in the course objectives: "The HBSE sequence of courses shall consider and promote student understanding of **how to reframe deficit-based theoretical and practice models to reflect a strengths-based expression of client systems . . .**" (Boldface in original.)
Comparative Perspectives	Stated in the HBSE sequence goal and outcome measures: "The overarching goal of the HBSE course sequence is to enable *students to critically analyze and understand human behavior and development from multiple theoretical perspectives. . . This lens of informed sensitive analysis then facilitates the student's ability to select from a broader range of theoretical and practice perspectives. . . which promote empathic and empowering relationships. . .*"
Logical Flow	The first few class sessions present students with a framework for understanding and interpreting theory. Each subsequent session focuses on a set of related theoretical perspectives, including systems, behavioral, social psychological, social learning, and psychodynamic theories.
Diversity	Each class session includes content on the theory's "strengths and limitations across systems, contexts, and settings." Unfortunately, little other detail is available about integration of diversity content.
Theory for Practice	Students are asked to complete two interviews and relate interview findings to the literature. Additionally, the final includes a theory-for-practice component in which students apply theory to a case.
Outline of Weekly Topics	1. Overview of the course 2. The Nature of Theory 3. Systems and ecological theory 4. The social context of development 5. Perspectives on lifespan development 6. Psychodynamic Theory 7. Symbolic interactionism 8. Humanistic and existential perspectives 9. Behavioral and social learning theory 10. Cognitive and moral development 11. The strengths perspective 12. Empowerment perspectives 13. Exam 14. Summary and Review

APPENDIX 4. Systems-Oriented HB&SE Course (Vanderbeek, 2002)

Criteria	How Met
Reciprocal Relationships	Stated in the course goals: "To apply on ecological systems perspective to *understanding mutual effects that individuals and larger systems have upon each other*, including social and economic forces, in either promoting (empowering) or deterring people from achieving optimal health and well-being."
Lifespan	Outlined in the course description: "Overview of theoretical perspectives applied to understanding biopsychosocial dimensions of the person, *individual behavior and development throughout the lifespan*, and within contexts of diversities of family, group, community, organizational, and cultural systems."
Systems	Outlined in the course description: "Overview of theoretical perspectives applied to understanding biopsychosocial dimensions of the person, individual behavior and development throughout the lifespan, and *within contexts of diversities of family, group, community, organizational, and cultural systems.*"
Well-Being	Stated in the course goals: "To apply an ecological systems perspective along with other course content to identify strengths of various social systems, as well as environmental obstacles to *their optimal health, well-being, and empowerment throughout the life cycle.*" This is reiterated in the academic outcomes: "To analyze how theory and knowledge presented in this course *fit with strengths-based practice and empowerment of individuals and larger social systems.*"
Comparative Perspectives	Stated in the course goals: "To develop theoretical foundations for practice by *applying critical thinking skills to knowledge and theory of human behavior.*" It is reiterated in the academic outcomes: "*To critically analyze and apply knowledge of bio-psycho-social variables that affect individual development.*"
Logical Flow	The course focuses on systems in decreasing size, beginning with culture and community then ending with families and individuals.
Diversity	Stated topics, required readings, and class activities for most class meetings include content that relates concepts to human differences in race, ethnicity, culture, gender, sexual orientation, and/or class.
Theory for Practice	In-class activities include application of theory to case studies. Little detailed information is available about at-home assignments.
Outline for Weekly Topics	1. Introduction and overview of the course 2. Introduction to theory 3. Introduction to culture and cultural competence 4. Exam and discussion of final paper 5. Self assessment 6. Communities 7. Small towns and neighborhoods 8. Organizations 9. Organizational culture 10. Groups 11. Groups and Families 12. Exam and discussion of family diversity 13. Traditional theories of the lifespan 14. Alternative theories of the lifespan 15. Traditional models of moral development

APPENDIX 5. Systems-Oriented HB&SE Course Meeting Mulroy and Austin (2004) Framework Criteria (Reed, 2002)

Criteria		How Met
Social Justice–Redistribution of rights, resources, and power and amelioration of structural inequalities.		Stated in the course description: "There is a focus on oppression, discrimination, prejudice, and privilege *and their relationship to social and economic justice* for populations served by social workers." This is reiterated in the course objectives, and three class sessions focus on social justice.
Political Economy–Exploration of the complex, interdependent relationship between politics and economy in communities and larger societies, including the impact of globalization.		Stated in the course description: "This course examines theory and research knowledge about *political, economic, and societal structures and* processes related to communities, groups, and organizations within contemporary society."
Social Problems–Macro-level problems that are documented objectively through facts that attest to their persistence and/or growth over time. There must also be a perception shared by many people that these problems should be addressed.		Stated in the course objectives: "*Identify, describe, and discuss the role of risk and protective social factors in relation to social problems,* social work interventions and social/economic justice."
Social Policies–A formally organized collective response to a social problem, usually developed and managed by government bodies and/or agencies.		One class session explicitly addresses the relationship of social work theory and public policy.
Collective Responses–Non-governmental and/or less formally organized collaborative efforts to address the effects of social problems and policies and seek solutions toward social change.		Stated in the instructor's notes on teaching philosophy: "*A major goal [of this course] is to develop the knowledge to think, plan, problem-solve, and create change at larger systems levels,* and to understand how larger systems impact individuals, families, and groups."
Structure–Includes the components of these systems and their relationships to one another within the system.	**Communities**–i.e., the specific constellation of merchants, schools, public services, etc.	Each of these topics is discussed in more than one class session, and readings clearly include material on both the structure and process of communities, organizations, and groups.
	Organizations–i.e., size, distribution of employees and work	
	Groups–i.e., membership & leadership	
Process–Includes the interactions of these components as they work towards their objectives.	**Communities**–i.e., type and degree of collaboration between entities	
	Organizations–i.e., type of relations between line staff and management	
	Groups–i.e., selection of leaders and members	

APPENDIX 5 (continued)

Criteria	How Met	
Outline of Weekly Topics	1. Outline of the course, introductions 2. Introductions to macro knowledge areas 3. introduction to community, organization, inter-organizational theory, and culture 4. Social justice, stratifications, privilege, power, oppression, and diversity 5. Organizations continued 6. Community and society continued 7. Public policy and social work theory 8. Comparisons/uses of paradigms & theories	9. Diversity and groups continued 10. Organizations and society continued 11. Social work in community and society–application of concepts & theories 12. Working in organizations 13. Applying theory and knowledge to working for social justice 14. Review and discuss models in relation to social justice, social change, and muticultural issues

Social Work Textbooks on Human Behavior and the Social Environment: An Analysis of the Social Environment Component

Sarah Taylor
Elizabeth A. Mulroy
Michael J. Austin

SUMMARY. This analysis of fourteen foundation frequently used Human Behavior and Social Environment (HB&SE) textbooks is based on the Council on Social Work Education's (2001) guidelines for HB&SE and a framework for integrating content related to the social environment. Specific criteria for assessment included how well the textbook reflected the reciprocal nature of human behavior and the social environment, presented a strengths perspective, incorporated diversity content, and covered material related to families, groups, organizations, communities and political economy. Three types of HB&SE textbooks were

---

Sarah Taylor, MSW, is Doctoral Research Assistant and Michael J. Austin, PhD, (E-mail: mjaustin@uclink4.Berkeley.edu) is Professor, School of Social Welfare, University of California, Berkeley. Elizabeth A. Mulroy, PhD, is Associate Professor, School of Social Work, University of Maryland-Baltimore.

[Haworth co-indexing entry note]: "Social Work Textbooks on Human Behavior and the Social Environment: An Analysis of the Social Environment Component." Taylor, Sarah, Elizabeth A. Mulroy, and Michael J. Austin. Co-published simultaneously in *Journal of Human Behavior in the Social Environment* (The Haworth Social Work Practice Press, an imprint of The Haworth Press, Inc.) Vol. 10, No. 3, 2004, pp. 85-109; and: *The Conundrum of Human Behavior in the Social Environment* (ed: Marvin D. Feit and John S. Wodarski) The Haworth Social Work Practice Press, an imprint of The Haworth Press, Inc., 2004,pp. 85-109. Single or multiple copies of this article are available for a fee from The Haworth Document Delivery Service [1-800-HAWORTH, 9:00 a.m. - 5:00 p.m. (EST). E-mail address: docdelivery@haworthpress.com].

© 2004 by The Haworth Press, Inc. All rights reserved.
Digital Object Identifier: 10.1300/J137v10n03_04

identified (*life cycle, systems,* and *theory*), and results are presented by textbook type. The findings suggest that increased attention to content related to the macro social environment and to the inter-relationships of macro, meso, and micro forces would strengthen HB&SE texts. *[Article copies available for a fee from The Haworth Document Delivery Service: 1-800-HAWORTH. E-mail address: <docdelivery@haworthpress.com> Website: <http://www.HaworthPress.com> © 2004 by The Haworth Press, Inc. All rights reserved.]*

KEYWORDS. Social work textbooks, social environment component, human behavior textbooks, social environment textbooks, HB&SE textbooks

INTRODUCTION

As the Human Behavior and Social Environment (HB&SE) content in the social work curriculum has evolved from psychoanalytically focused material taught by faculty outside the social work department to one of five CSWE-required curriculum content areas in accredited schools of social work, there has been a growth in the number of social work textbooks designed specifically to support HB&SE courses. The texts vary widely in focus, scope, and topics covered, much like the diversity of the HB&SE courses (Taylor, Mulroy, & Austin, 2004).

Despite the critical role of HB&SE in the social work curriculum, little research has been done on the required courses or the texts used. This analysis includes a review of fourteen frequently used HB&SE texts published between 1998-2003. In 1969, the CSWE began requiring that HB&SE include content on the social environment as well as on human behavior (Brooks, 1986). By 2001, the CSWE accreditation requirements had expanded to emphasize the *integration* of content on human behavior and the social environment in the HB&SE curriculum as noted below:

> Social work education programs provide content on the reciprocal relationships between human behavior and social environments. Content includes empirically based theories and knowledge that focus on the interactions between and among individuals, groups, societies, and economic systems. It includes theories and knowl-

edge of biological, sociological, cultural, psychological, and spiritual development across the life span; the range of social systems in which people live (individual, family, group, organizational, and community); and the ways social systems promote or deter people in maintaining or achieving health and well-being. (Council on Social Work Education, 2001, p. 35)

Because of the historical focus on human behavior in HB&SE courses and the evolving CSWE accreditation standards, this analysis includes an emphasis on social environment content as reflected in current textbooks.

BRIEF LITERATURE REVIEW

A review of research on graduate social work curriculum from 1975-1995 revealed only two empirical studies on HB&SE courses (Wodarski, Feit, & Green, 1995). Both studies were limited to very specific questions within the HB&SE curriculum. The Sutton (1981) study evaluated the effectiveness of using interactive versus didactic methods for teaching behavior theory with a two group pre-test, post-test design. The second study, Spero (1982), featured a one group pre-test, post-test design to determine how well students learned ego psychology (Wodarski et al., 1995). The authors of the review comment that, "... the field of teaching HB&SE content is ripe for further research" (p. 119).

The lack of research on HB&SE courses and texts is surprising given the perceived centrality of HB&SE in BSW curricula. In a survey of 147 BSW program directors, respondents ranked twenty-four of thirty HB&SE content items with an importance score of four or higher on a scale of five (Griffin & Eure, 1985). Further evidence of the value of HB&SE in BSW programs can be found in the shift from offering HBSE courses in education, psychology, or sociology courses outside of social work to courses offered inside the social work program. For example, Gibbs (1986) found that nearly 90% of HB&SE courses in BSW programs were being taught within the social work department (Gibbs, 1986). Gibbs notes that this is a major change from the early 1970s when a study by Stamm (1972) found that over 70% of social work departments did not teach their own HBSE courses (Gibbs, 1986).

There is some conflicting data about the effectiveness of HB&SE courses taught in social work departments versus HB&SE taught outside social work departments. A 1979 study comparing BSW students who took HB&SE in social work departments and students who took HB&SE through outside departments found no statistically significant differences between the students taking HBSE in or out of the department in terms of number of theoretical constructs taught, ability to apply theory to practice, or adoption of social work values (Sze, Keller, & Keller, 1979). However, a more recent study that compared MSW students taking HBSE in social work departments with graduate students in education taking HB&SE courses in education departments found that the students taking HB&SE in the social work department increased in their ability to perceive strengths in populations-at-risk while students taking HB&SE courses in the education department did not increase (Johnson & Rhodes, 2001). Clearly, further research on the effectiveness of HB&SE courses is required, particularly in light of evolving research on the nature of human behavior and the changing social environment.

Similar to the limited research on HB&SE, there has also been limited analysis of social work textbooks. A study of fourteen introductory social work texts of the 1970s that focused on social work as a profession and the field in general indicates that texts do express ideological content in implicit and explicit ways (Ephross & Reisch, 1982). The authors identified three ideological positions endorsed by the textbooks. Politically left of center texts located social problems in society and recommended social action to address these issues. "Centrist" texts either recognized social problems, but did not advocate for social change, or recognized social problems only to the extent that these problems affected social work with individuals and families. Politically right of center texts attributed social problems to individual flaws (Ephross & Reisch, 1982).

Though ideological content is not the focus of this analysis of textbooks, scholars commenting on HB&SE continue to debate how much attention should be given to human behavior and development in contrast to the constructs of the social environment. Whether or not textbook authors openly state their views on the HB vs. SE controversy, the organization, structure, and tone of their texts are likely to influence students' awareness and understanding of the social environment.

The specific questions we sought to answer through our analysis included:

- How are the texts structured?

- How is content on the social environment presented?
- How do the texts make the connection between theory and practice?
- How well do the texts fit with current CSWE curriculum standards?

METHOD OF ANALYSIS

Taylor, Austin, and Mulroy (2004) gathered 117 HB&SE course outlines for MSW classes from 60 schools of social work. Based on a scan of the outlines, a list of the most frequently cited texts was compiled. Fourteen texts were reviewed and are listed in Note 1.

The content analysis of each text included particular attention to the table of contents, preface, and content on the social environment. A fifteen-item assessment form was developed and applied to each text to guide the analysis and ensure consistency of data collected. Development of the form was based on the CSWE guidelines stated above as well as the Mulroy and Austin (2004) social environment framework discussed later in this article. The form included questions related to four areas:

1. General content including the structure of the text, audience, major themes, theory for practice emphasis.
2. General social environment content including the textbook's definition of the social environment and which structures of the social environment are discussed.
3. The extent of focus on social justice and social problems.
4. Specific social environment content including definitions of families, groups, organizations, and communities and amount of content on these concepts.

In order to document the breadth and depth of content on families, groups, organizations, and communities in the textbooks, we developed a list of sub-topics commonly covered for each construct of the social environment. For example, the family sub-topics list included: Functions of the family; families as systems; stages of family development; non-developmental crises (i.e., illness); family violence; racial, ethnic, and cultural diversity; gay, lesbian, bisexual, and transgender families; single-parent families; divorce; working with families; poverty; technology; and family policy. If a text had content on less than one-third of the sub-topics, we ranked it as "few topics covered." If it discussed between one-third and two-thirds of the sub-topics, it was rated as "many topics covered." If a text dealt with more than two-thirds of the sub-topics, it received a rating of "most topics covered."

There are several limitations to this analysis. While there was an extensive search of the literature for similar comparative analyses of HB&SE textbooks, none could be found even though they may exist. Second, there were insufficient financial and human resources to develop a comprehensive, in-depth assessment of each textbook. And third, the textbooks were assessed using the summaries prepared by one of the three co-authors, rather than using the complete books. While it is not known if this is the first comparative analysis of HB&SE textbooks, it is clear that further study of this key aspect of the social work curriculum is needed.

FINDINGS

Based on the analysis of the textbooks, the following three types of texts emerged: (1) individual or family life cycle textbooks, (2) *systems* textbooks, and (3) *theory* textbooks. Before describing the characteristics of each type of text, it should be noted that nearly all of the textbooks included human diversity content, discussed social problems, made some connections between human behavior and the social environment, and appeared to incorporate the CSWE accreditation guidelines. As a result, this analysis focuses more on the degree to which the social environment and related issues are integrated into the text, and the balance between human behavior and the social environment content.

The six *life cycle* textbooks reviewed include chapters that describe the developmental stages of individuals and/or families from birth through death. Some of these textbooks also include a section on various systems (groups, organizations, and communities), but the majority of the content emphasizes the life cycle. The strengths of these textbooks include their comprehensive coverage of human development, family issues, and the bio-psycho-social or ecological perspective as theory to inform social work practice. Based on the analysis of these six *life cycle* textbooks, there appears to be less attention given to groups, organizations, and communities. Their discussion of the social environment often focuses on how the individual experiences or is affected by groups, organizations, or communities, rather than treating these structures of the social environment as dynamic, interdependent systems. Their definitions of the social environment and its structures are frequently less explicit than the discussion found in the systems textbooks.

The *systems* textbooks tend to be organized around the concepts of the social environment, often with one or more separate chapters on individuals, families, groups, organizations, or communities. Most of the five *systems* textbooks reviewed also devote significant attention to the role of social justice issues, social work ethics and a broad array of social science theories. They provide explicit definitions of the social environment and its structures, with detailed content on groups, organizations, and communities. Individuals are often described as being one type or size of system, and all systems are described as interdependent entities irrespective of how individuals experience them. The s*ystems* textbooks also featured a greater emphasis on alternative perspectives, even though theories about human behavior were not explored in depth.

The third group of textbooks emphasized *multiple theories* such as systems theory, psychodynamic theory, and cognitive behavioral theory. The three *theory* textbooks in this analysis included detailed explanations of theoretical perspectives along with an emphasis on critical thinking skills needed for evaluating the usefulness of a given theory for social work practice and research. The *theory* textbooks varied in their treatment of the social environment, social work ethics, and social problems. The *theory* texts also tended to give less precise definitions of the social environment and its structures.

The data upon which the three clusters of textbooks are based can be found in Appendices 1-3. The structure of each figure follows the elements of the assessment form described in the methods section and the findings are noted in the form of brief statements. While each figure begins with general HB&SE content and the degree of emphasis on the social environment, it also includes brief descriptions of the specific social environment content and concludes with general impressions.

For example, Appendix 1 discusses the six *life cycle* textbooks. The main chapter headings of each text are given, as well as the texts' coverage of social justice and diversity issues, definition of the social environment, depth of content about families, groups, organizations, and communities, number of course outlines citing the text, and the reviewer's general impressions.

TOWARDS A FRAMEWORK FOR BUILDING THE SE COMPONENT OF HB&SE

As described in the introduction, the focus of our analysis of HB&SE textbooks is the incorporation of SE concepts into the HB&SE curriculum, especially since the course content typically favors HB over SE (Brooks, 1986).

Mulroy and Austin (2004) present a framework for selecting and organizing course content (see Figure 1) related to the social environment. Their framework suggests that four primary forces of the macro social environment (social justice, political economy, social problems, and social policy) influence community, organizational, and group dynamics. The impact of the macro social environment can be mediated by collective responses–the collaborative efforts of groups, organizations, and communities to address these forces. The figure illustrates that as the horizontal and vertical linkages between these entities are constantly in flux, and as the societal forces change, the landscape of the social environment shifts. This framework seeks to capture the complex social environment of modern society, where a constellation of social forces can shape the array of social, political, and economic relations in communities and nations of all sizes. The concepts in the framework are defined in Figure 2.

FIGURE 1. Mulroy and Austin (2004) Social Environment Framework Criteria

Social Justice–Redistribution of rights, resources, and power and amelioration of structural inequalities.	
Political Economy–Exploration of the complex, interdependent relationship between politics and economy in communities and larger societies, including the impact of globalization.	
Social Problems–Macro-level problems that are documented objectively through facts that attest to their persistence and/or growth over time. There must also be a perception shared by many people that these problems should be addressed.	
Social Policies–A formally organized collective response to a social problem, usually developed and managed by governmental bodies and/or agencies.	
Collective Responses–Non-governmental and/or less formally organized collaborative efforts to address the effects of social problems and policies and seek solutions toward social change.	
Structure–Includes the components of these systems and their relationships to one another within the system	**Communities**–i.e., specific constellation of merchants, schools, public services, etc.
	Organizations–i.e., size, distribution of employees, and work
	Groups–i.e., membership & leadership
Process–Includes the interactions of these components as they work towards their objectives	**Communities**–i.e., type and degree of collaboration between entities
	Organizations–i.e., type of relations between line staff and management
	Groups–i.e., selection of leaders and members

FIGURE 2. Application of Mulroy and Austin (2004) SE Framework to Systems Texts

		Hutchison (2003b)	Kirst-Ashman (2000)	Longres (2000)	Pillari & Newsome (1998)	Schriver (2001)
Social Justice–Redistribution of rights, resources, and power and amelioration of structural inequalities.		X	X	X	X	X
Political Economy–Exploration of the complex, interdependent relationship between politics and economy in communities and larger societies, including the impact of globalization.		X	X			X
Social Problems–Macro-level problems that are documented objectively through facts that attest to their persistence and/or growth over time. There must also be a perception shared by many people that these problems should be addressed.		X	X	X	X	X
Social Policies–A formally organized collective response to a social problem, usually developed and managed by governmental bodies and/or agencies.		X	X			
Collective Responses–Non-governmental and/or less formally organized collaborative efforts to address the effects of social problems and policies and seek solutions toward social change		X	X			X
Structure–Includes the components of these systems and their relationships to one another within the system.	Communities–i.e., the specific constellation of merchants, schools, public services, etc.	X	X	X	X	X
	Organizations–i.e., size, distribution of employees and work	X	X	X	X	X
	Groups–i.e., membership & leadership	X	X	X	X	X
Process–Includes the interactions of these components as they work towards their objectives.	Communities–i.e., type and degree of collaboration between entities	X	X	X	X	X
	Organizations–i.e., type of relations between line staff and management	X	X	X	X	X
	Groups–i.e., selection of leaders and members	X	X	X	X	X

We applied this social environment framework to the five systems texts described in the preceding section. Though many lifespan and theory texts include material on the social environment, we used the framework to evaluate primarily the systems texts because their objective, whether stated implicitly or explicitly, is to structure and organize content on the social environment. We used a similar methodology for developing and applying the framework criteria to the texts as we did for the CSWE guideline-based criteria described above. First, we defined the criteria based on the Mulroy and Austin (2004) framework. Then, all three authors rated each of the five texts using the summaries prepared in the initial stage of analysis using a checklist of the framework criteria. Two of the three raters re-reviewed the texts themselves along with the summaries to ensure a fair and accurate assessment. The results are noted in Figure 2.

Our major finding was that while all systems texts adequately covered material related to the concepts of groups, organizations, and communities, only two of the five texts provided substantial content in each of the macro concepts: Social justice, political economy, social problems, social policies, and collective responses. This mirrors the results in our analysis of HB&SE course outlines, in which coverage of the concepts related to groups, organizations, and communities was strong, but concepts related to the macro social environment were less adequately addressed (Taylor et al., 2004). No doubt these findings are related, as there is an inter-dependent relationship between course content and textbook content.

CONCLUSION

This study provided the opportunity to examine fourteen current HBSE textbooks widely in use in MSW social work education programs. Of particular interest was the extent to which these textbooks responded to CSWE accreditation requirements (2001) in terms of the *reciprocal* relationships between human behavior and social environments, with an emphasis on scope and treatment of the social environment as a concept. We conclude that the majority of textbooks approached the subject from either a *life cycle*, *systems*, or *theory* perspective. The *systems* textbooks emphasized definitions of the social environment and its structures more than those reflecting a *life cycle* or *theory* perspective. For example, the *systems* textbooks gave more emphasis to the structure and process of groups, organizations, and local communities; social justice; and social problems. However, they gave less attention to the concepts of political economy, social policies, and collective responses.

One question that emerges from this study is: Do faculty members select a major textbook that corresponds to their own syllabus, or is a syllabus created from the substance and content of the selected textbook? If the latter is the case, then textbook authors face a special challenge in seeking to successfully *integrate* material on human behavior and the social environment that is also *reciprocal* (i.e., both a unified whole and equivalent) This study suggests that having a clear conceptualization of what constitutes the social environment is a place to start. For example, as noted in some texts, rapid technological changes, the global economy, and shifting public policy priorities have created rapid and large-scale changes at the local as well as state and national levels that are now a part of the social environmental. Based on this review of current HB&SE textbooks, it is clear that more attention is needed to link the different aspects of the social environment in order for students to fully understand their dynamic interaction. First, the macro societal forces are clearly impacting the dynamics of groups, organizations, and communities (Mulroy & Austin, 2004). Second, there is a need to link together social environment concepts such as poverty, social justice, diversity, and empowerment. As Craig points out, "when people or areas suffer from a combination of linked problems such as unemployment, poor skills, low-incomes, poor housing, high crime environments, bad health, and family breakdown," they create a powerful context that impacts many of the recipients of social services (Craig, 2002, p. 672). An understanding of HB&SE requires a weaving together of these broad elements in the social environment with the principles of social justice in order to see the "ways social systems promote or deter people in maintaining or achieving health and well-being." (Council on Social Work Education, 2001, p. 35). To the extent that HB&SE textbooks address the interactive nature of all of these elements in the social environment, they will help to further (1) the *integration* of human behavior *and* the social environment, and (2) the *reciprocal relationship* or wholeness of understanding human behavior *in* the social environment.

NOTE 1: LIST OF TEXTS REVIEWED

Ashford, J., Lecroy, C., & Lortie, K. (2001). *Human Behavior in the Social Environment: A Multidimensional Perspective*. Belmont, CA: Wadsworth/Thompson Learning.

Bloom, M., & Klein, W. (Eds.). (1997). *Controversial Issues in Human Behavior in the Social Environment*. Boston, MA: Allyn and Bacon.

Germain, C., & Bloom, M. (1999). *Human Behavior in the Social Environment: An Ecological View*. New York: Columbia University Press.

Greene, R. (Ed.). (1999). *Human Behavior Theory and Social Work Practice*. New York: Aldine de Gruyter.

Hutchison, E. (2003a). *Dimensions of Human Behavior: The Changing Life Course*. Thousand Oaks, CA: Sage Publications.

Hutchison, E. (2003b). *Dimensions of Human Behavior: Person and Environment*. Thousand Oaks, CA: Sage Publications.

Kirst-Ashman, K. (2000). *Human Behavior, Communities, Organizations, and Groups in the Macro Social Environment: An Empowerment Approach*. Belmont, CA: Wads- worth/Thompson Learning.

Longres, J. (2000). *Human Behavior in the Social Environment*. Belmont, CA: Wadsworth/Thompson Learning.

Pillari, V., & Newsome, M. (1998). *Human Behavior in the Social Environment: Families, Groups, Organizations, and Communities*. Pacific Grove, CA: Brooks/Cole Publishing Company.

Robbins, S., Chatterjee, P., & Canda, E. (1998). *Contemporary Human Behavior Theory: A Critical Perspective for Social Work*. Boston, MA: Allyn and Bacon.

Saleebey, D. (2001). *Human Behavior and Social Environments: A Biopsychosocial Approach*. New York: Columbia University Press.

Schriver, J. (2001). *Human Behavior and the Social Environment: Shifting Paradigms in Essential Knowledge for Social Work Practice*. Boston, MA: Allyn and Bacon.

Urdang, E. (2002). *Human Behavior in the Social Environment: Interweaving the Inner and Outer Worlds*. New York: The Haworth Social Work Practice Press.

Zastrow, C., & Kirst-Ashman, K. (2004). *Understanding Human Behavior and the Social Environment*. Belmont, CA: Wadsworth/Thompson Learning.

REFERENCES

Brooks, W. (1986). Human behavior/social environment: Past and present, future or folly? *Journal of Social Work Education*, 22(1), 18-23.

Council on Social Work Education. (2001). *Handbook of Accreditation Standards and Procedures*. Alexandria, VA.

Ephross, P., & Reisch, M. (1982). The ideology of some social work texts. *The Social Service Review*, 56(2), 273-291.

Gibbs, P. (1986). HBSE in the undergraduate curriculum: A survey. *Journal of Social Work Education*, 22(2), 46-52.

Griffin, J., & Eure, G. (1985). Defining the professional foundation in social work education. *Journal of Social Work Education*, 21(3), 73-91.

Johnson, M., & Rhodes, R. (2001). "Give me strengths!" Evaluating the effectiveness of a graduate level HBSE course. *Journal of Human Behavior in the Social Environment*, 4(1), 1-18.

Mulroy, E., & Austin, M. (2004). Towards a comprehensive framework for understanding the social environment: In search of theory for practice. *Journal of Human Behavior in the Social Environment*, 10(3), 25-59.

Sze, W. Keller, R., & Keller, D. (1979). A comparative study of two different teaching and curricular arrangements in human behavior and social environment. *Journal of Education for Social Work, 15*(1), 103-109.

Taylor, S., Mulroy, E., & Austin, M. (2004). Evaluating the social environment component of human behavior and the social environment. *Journal of Human Behavior in the Social Environment, 10*(3), 61-84.

Wodarski, J., Feit, M., & Green, R. (1995). Graduate social work education: A review of two decades of empirical research and considerations for the future. *The Social Service Reveiw, 69*(1), 108-130.

APPENDIX 1. General Description of Life Cycle HB&SE Textbooks

	Ashford, J., LeCroy, C., & Lortie, K. (2001)	Germain, C. & Bloom, M. (1999)	Hutchison, E. (2003a)
Text Structure	This 638 page text is divided into 12 chapters. Because chapter 4 deals specifically with the social dimension, its topic headings are listed here: *Defining the family *Family life cycle *Groups as social subsystems *Support systems *Contexts: Communities, organizations, and institutions *Racial and ethnic considerations *Gender and sexism *Social hazards The remaining chapters present a lifespan model.	This 472 page text is divided into 2 parts. Because Part I deals specifically with the social dimension, its chapters are listed here: *The Ecological Perspective *Society, Culture, Community, & the Physical Environment *Complex Organizations *Schools and Work Sites *Small Groups *Families *Genetics/Biology Part II presents a family life cycle model.	Companion text to the author's systems text. This 551 page text is divided into 10 chapters, organized into nine stages of the lifespan, from conception through very late adulthood. (Chapter one provides an introduction to the life course perspective.) Each chapter begins with case studies and ends with implications for SW and reflection questions.
Audience	BSW, MSW	Not specifically identified.	Not specifically identified.
Theory Explication	Ecological approach emphasized	Ecological approach is emphasized.	Ecological approach and life course perspective emphasized, but other theories are compared and contrasted with these perspectives in an excellent table on pg. 45. Also, theories are introduced as relevant to material in each chapter (i.e., attachment theory is discussed in chapter on infancy.)
Major Themes	*biopsychosocial model *developmental issues *integration of community and social issues into developmental stages.	*to integrate information about person and environment without overwhelming the student.	*to help social work students learn to apply general social science knowledge in the specific social work situations they encounter.
Theory for Practice	Little direct reference	Little direct reference	The "implications" sections in each chapter include bulleted lists of practice suggestions and skill-building questions for practice based on the information presented in the chapter.
Definition of the Social Environment	The authors cite Nurcombe & Gallagher (1986): "The social dimension refers to the systems of social relationships that a person interacts with individually or in a group." (p. 30)	Not clearly defined.	A figure in chapter one (pg. 20) explains the components of the social environment that influence individuals.

	Ashford, J., LeCroy, C., & Lortie, K. (2001)	Germain, C. & Bloom, M. (1999)	Hutchison, E. (2003a)
Structures of the Social Environment	"...families, communities, other support systems, gay and lesbian relationships, cultural groups, ethnic groups, and social institutions such as churches, political parties, schools, and health care and welfare institutions." (p. 30)	"Social settings comprise the world of other human beings. Its components include pairs or dyads . . . families; neighborhoods, enclaves (Abrahamson, 1996), and communities; natural groups and social (formed) networks. The social environment also includes formal organizations . . . religious organizations; political and economic structures ... and social space and social time." (p. 33)	The structures presented in the figure on pg. 20 include social movements, communities, formal organizations, small groups, families, dyads, the physical environment, social institutions and social structure, and culture.

SE in Life Cycle HB&SE Textbooks

	Ashford, J., LeCroy, C., & Lortie, K. (2001)	Germain, C. & Bloom, M. (1999)	Hutchison, E. (2003a)
Social Problems & Societal Focus	Social problems are discussed mainly through the individual case narratives. Many narratives "deal with racism, poverty, sexual orientation, youth, ageism, and other topics related to the impact of human diversity on development."	Social problems are given less focus, with the exception of chapter two, which highlights the experiences of a variety of marginalized populations, such as individuals who identify as gay or lesbian, migrant workers, & immigrants.	Social problems are discussed both through individual case narratives and in the main body of the text. Poverty, welfare reform, issues related to immigration, and community violence are among the social problems highlighted. Human diversity issues are discussed throughout the text.
Social Justice & Social Work Values	The code is not cited in the introduction, and little reference is made to specific social work values.	The code is not cited in the introduction, and little reference is made to specific social work values.	The code is not cited in the introduction, and little reference is made to specific social work values.
Family– Definition and # of topics covered.	"Most discussions about the family include two related aspects of family: the family as 'headquarters for human development' and the family as a social institution." (p. 109). Covers many topics.	They identify two "categories" of family: One being the family tied by blood and marriage bonds, the other by the "current family constellation (structure) in which people have chosen to live." (p. 155) Covers many topics.	In the chapter on conception, pregnancy, and childbirth, a two-page section describes the plurality of family in modern life and indicated that a definition of family must take this diversity into account. Covers few topics.
Groups– Definition and # of topics covered.	Outlines eight features of groups: Communication, influence, interaction, interdependence, interrelations, psychological significance, shared identity, and structure. (p.113) Covers many topics.	Not clearly stated. Covers many topics.	Not clearly stated. Few topics covered.

APPENDIX 1 (continued)

	Ashford, J., LeCroy, C., & Lortie, K. (2001)	Germain, C. & Bloom, M. (1999)	Hutchison, E. (2003a)
Organizations– Definition and # of topics covered.	"A formal organization is any large social group that is designed to achieve specific objectives rationally." (p. 126) Covers few topics.	Not clearly stated. Covers few topics.	Not clearly stated. Few topics covered.
Community– Definition and # of topics covered.	Not clearly stated. Covers few topics.	Not clearly stated. Covers few topics.	Not clearly stated. Few topics covered.
Number of syllabi citing text	19	17	7
Impressions	Seems most appropriate for readers with a limited social science background.	Strong HB focus with thorough explanation of systems theory.	Strong HB focus with a wealth of material.

General Description of Life Cycle HB&SE Textbooks

	Saleebey, D. (2001)	Urdang, E. (2002)	Zastrow, C. & Kirst-Ashman, K. (2004)
Text Structure	This 509 page text is divided into 13 chapters: *Introduction *Meaning-Making *Strengths and Resilience *Biopsychosocial Understanding *Nature and Nurture, Neurons and Narratives: Putting it All Together *2 chapters on theory *5 chapters on family life cycle *Reprise, Vision, and the Final Conversation	This 642 page text is divided into four parts: *The Biopsychosocial Perspective *The Life Cycle *Special Issues *Integration Because Part I deals with the social environment, its chapters are listed here: *Overview *2 theory chapters *Social Systems and the Community, Culture, and Diversity *2 chapters on family Each chapter ends with learning exercises.	This 644 page text is divided into four parts: *Infancy and Childhood *Adolescence and Young Adulthood *Middle Adulthood *Later Adulthood Each part includes separate chapters on how biological, psychological, and social systems impact the individual at a given life stage. Though there are not separate chapters on families, small groups, organizations, and communities, these topics are dealt with in the introductory chapter and revisited in the social systems chapters of each part.
Audience	MSW, PhD	MSW–year-long HBSE	BSW, MSW
Theory Explication	Ecological approach is emphasized, but psychodynamic & cognitive also presented.	Use of psychodynamic theory within biopsychosocial framework is emphasized.	The text emphasizes systems theory, but highlights other theories throughout. For example, Part III, on middle adulthood, describes conflict, functionalist, and interactionist perspectives.

	Saleebey, D. (2001)	Urdang, E. (2002)	Zastrow, C. & Kirst-Ashman, K. (2004)
Major Themes	*critical thinking *social justice *hope *strengths perspective, *understanding the contexts in which humans grow and develop	*The inner world of clients –author comments that she expects social environment to be taught in second semester of year-long HBSE sequence.	*the biopsychosocial perspective *interactions among human and social systems *communicating social work values *well-being *social justice
Theory for Practice	Little direct reference.	The learning exercises at the end of each chapter emphasize critical thinking and application of theory to practice situations.	Social work roles for intervention are highlighted throughout. There is an excellent section in the social systems middle adulthood chapter that teaches students how to create and use EcoMaps to assess family systems. There is also a helpful text box on page 469 that teaches specific questions for assessing a human service organization.
Definition of the Social Environment	Not clearly defined. Saleebey cites Brofenbrenner's (1989) four levels of socialenvironment: Micro, mezzo, exo, macro. (pp. 148-149).	Not clearly defined.	"... the social environment involves the conditions, circumstances, and human interactions that encompass human beings." (p. 7)
Structures of the Social Environment	*micro = face-to-face interactions *mezzo = interactions of micro systems *exo = systems that affect individuals, but in which many individuals do not participate (i.e., school boards) *macro = systems responsible for creation of social policy and ideology.	This is also not defined specifically, but the sub-headings under the "Social Environment" topic area in chapter four include: Economic, employment, public school education, and communities, organizations, and social issues. The text also includes two chapters on family.	In figures on pages 12-13, the authors explain the interactions of the individual with various social systems, including families, groups, institutions, organizations, cultures, and communities as well as social forces.
Social Problems & Societal Focus	Social problems are highlighted throughout the text, both from current events, and through discussion of specific social problems in general. Human diversity issues are woven seamlessly into the text.	The social issues section includes discussion of discrimination & prejudice, violence, imprisonment, incarceration of the mentally ill, and substance abuse. There is also a separate chapter on culture and diversity.	Social problems are highlighted throughout, both through discussion in the body of the text of topics such as HIV, ethnocentrism, and sexism, but also through text boxes featuring narratives of how social problems impact individuals. Human diversity issues are discussed throughout.

APPENDIX 1 (continued): SE in Life Cycle HB&SE Textbooks

	Saleebey, D. (2001)	Urdang, E. (2002)	Zastrow, C. & Kirst-Ashman, K. (2004)
Social Justice & Social Work Values	Saleebey highlights two ethical focus areas that echo the values described in the code: strengths/ hope and battling oppression.	The code is not cited in the introduction, and little reference is made to specific social work values.	Several chapters include case examples that present ethical dilemmas; for example, a two-page text box in Chapter 2 discusses ethical issues for social workers involved in abortion counseling.
Family– Definition and # of topics covered.	Saleebey quotes Hartman and Laird (1983): "[a family] consists of two or more people who have made a commitment to share living space, have developed close emotional ties, and share a variety of family roles and functions." (p. 265) Covers most topics.	Not clearly stated. Covers many topics.	The authors quote Barker (1999): "A family is a primary group. This entails 'people who are intimate and have frequent face-to-face contact with one another, have norms ... in common and share mutually enduring and extensive influences.'" (p. 130) Covers many topics.
Groups– Definition and # of topics covered.	Not clearly stated. Covers few topics.	Not clearly stated. Covers few topics. Some discussion of self help groups: "Self-help groups–people with common problems who meet to provide mutual support and informal education–have proliferated in recent years." (p. 135)	The authors quote Johnson & Johnson (1997): ". . . two or more individuals in face-to-face interaction, each aware of his or her membership in the group, each aware of the others who belong to the group, and each aware of their positive interdependence as they strive to achieve mutual goals." (p. 315). Covers most topics.
Organizations– Definition and # of topics covered.	Not clearly stated. Covers few topics.	Not clearly stated. Some discussion of SW organizations. Covers few topics.	Authors quote Daft (1998): "Organizations are '(1) social entities that (2) are goal directed, (3) are designed as deliberately structured and coordinated activity systems, and (4) are linked to the external environment.'" (p. 23) Covers many topics.
Community - Definition and # of topics covered.	Not clearly stated. Covers few topics.	Not clearly stated. Covers few topics.	Authors quote Homan (1999): "A community is 'a number of people who have something in common with one another that connects them in some way and that distinguishes them from others.'" (p. 12-13) Covers many topics.

	Saleebey, D. (2001)	Urdang, E. (2002)	Zastrow, C. & Kirst-Ashman, K. (2004)
Number of syllabi citing text	2	2	17 (Count is for 2001 version)
Impressions	Deals with complex issues. Seems most appropriate for students with some social science background.	Seems appropriate for readers with social science background and interest in mental health.	Excellent balance of HB & SE and theory & practice.

APPENDIX 2. General Description of Systems HB&SE Textbooks

	Hutchison, E. (2003b)	Kirst-Ashman, K. (2000)	Longres, J. (2000)
Text Structure	Companion systems text to author's life course text. This 640 page text is divided into three parts: I. Intro to HBSE theories and ideas II. Person III. Environment The chapters in Part III include: *The physical environment *Culture *Social Institutions and Social Structure *Families *Small groups *Formal organizations *Communities *Social Movements Each part begins with a visual essay & each chapter ends with implications for SW & reflection questions.	Author recommends this systems text to accompany Zastrow & Kirst-Ashman (2004). This 283 page text is divided into twelve chapters: *Introduction *Community Theory *Human Behavior, Power, & Empowerment *Neighborhood Empowerment *Theory about Orgs. *The Internal and External Environments of Orgs. *HB in Traditional Org. Env. *HB and Empowerment in Orgs. *Empowerment of People with DD in Community and Org. Environments *Types of Groups *HB in Groups: Theories *Conclusion	This 596 page text is divided into five parts: *A Critical Perspective on Social Systems *Communities in Society *Family Life *Large and Small Groups (includes content on organizations) *Individual Development Across the Life Span Each chapter ends with a section on implications for practice and discussion questions.
Audience	Not specifically identified.	BSW, MSW	Not specifically identified.

APPENDIX 2 (continued)

	Hutchison, E. (2003b)	Kirst-Ashman, K. (2000)	Longres, J. (2000)
Theory Explication	Chapter 2 presents systems, conflict, rational choice, social constructionist, psychodynamic, developmental, social behavioral, and humanistic theories. The chapter summarizes how the perspectives rank in terms of clarity, testability, diversity, comprehensiveness, and usefulness in a chart on page 50. The content is organized by theoretical explanations of concepts, with minor theories identified as fitting in with the major theories using sidebar notes.	Emphasizes ecological systems theory. In each of the chapters focused on theory (one each for communities, organizations, and groups), the author summarizes major points of various theoretical perspectives.	The text emphasizes the systems approach. Part IV, on groups and organizations, includes two chapters on broad theories to enhance understanding of group dynamics such as structural functionalism and symbolic interactionism. Part V, on individual development, also introduces psychological theories—psychodynamic, cognitive, and developmental perspectives.
Major Themes	*a holistic understanding of HB * breadth over depth *helps students apply general knowledge to unique situations	"empowerment, diversity, populations-at-risk, and the promotion of social and economic justice... critical thinking, spirituality, and ethical issues." (p. xix)	*diversity *populations-at-risk *social and economic justice.
Theory for Practice	The "implications" sections in each chapter include bulleted lists of practice suggestions and skill-building questions for practice based on the information presented in the chapter.	The pull-out text boxes provide examples of theory applied to social work settings and/or cases.	The implications for practice and the discussion question sections at the end of each chapter encourage students to think critically and to apply theory.
Definition of the Social Environment	Not clearly stated. Uses levels focus: micro, mezzo, exo, macro.	"... the sum total of social and cultural conditions, circumstances, and human interactions that encompass human beings." (p. 5)	"The social environment consists of the personal and impersonal relations surrounding individuals and social systems." (p. 52)
Structures of the Social Environment	*The physical environment *Culture *Social Institutions & Structure *Families *Small groups *Formal organizations *Communities *Social Movements	In macro social environment: *Community *Neighborhood *Organization *Group	"It includes the individual as a system and the social systems—the other persons and the groups, families, communities, organizations, societies, and nations—with which the individual interacts and which directly or indirectly influence the individual's behavior and development." (p.52)

SE in Systems HB&SE Textbooks

	Hutchison, E. (2003b)	Kirst-Ashman, K. (2000)	Longres, J. (2000)
Social Problems & Societal Focus	The text is attentive to demographic trends that influence practice, such as an increase in immigration & the aging of the population. Human diversity content is incorporated throughout. Chapter 9 highlights inequality.	Social problems and human diversity are highlighted throughout the text. Plus Chapter 9 comments on the empowerment of persons with DD, and Chapter 12 applies concepts to various populations-at-risk.	About 2/3 of the text is devoted to social problems and social issues. A wide range of social problems are discussed throughout the text including poverty, racism, homophobia, shifting demographics, public policy, and anomie.
Social Justice & Social Work Values	The chapter on social movements addresses the role of social workers in social justice movements. Maintains that SWs must seek a balance between activism and professionalism.	In Chapter 1, Kirst-Ashman cites the NASW code of ethics in a special section titled, "Promotion of Social and Economic Justice." The author emphasizes equitable distribution of resources.	The emphasis on social justice and on helping students to develop social work values is made clear throughout the text. In chapter three, the NASW code of ethics is excerpted in a text box.
Family—Definition and # of topics covered.	Hutchison quotes the NASW (1981): "a grouping that consists of two or more individuals who define themselves as a family and who over time assume those obligations to one another that are generally considered an essential component of family systems." (p. 411). Covers many topics.	Not included in text.	Author comments that ". . . family is difficult to define...As popularly used, family has connotations about the quality or nature of the relationship. . . The term is also used to apply to the activities, socializing activities, nursing and protective activities, materially helpful activities, or consumption activities." (pp. 204-205). Covers most topics.
Groups—Definition and # of topics covered.	". . . a collection of individuals who interact with each other, perceive themselves as belonging to a group, are interdependent, join together to accomplish a goal or fulfill a need through joint association, and are influenced by a set of rules or norms." (p. 437) Covers most topics.	Author quotes Barker (1995): "a collection of people, brought together by mutual interests, who are capable of consistent and uniform action." (p. 6) Covers most topics. Focus on task groups.	"Groups are human systems in which the members are interdependent and share an identity. . . In small groups, members are interdependent and influence each other through face-to-face interaction." (p. 330) Covers many topics.
Organizations—Definition and # of topics covered.	Hutchison cites Bozeman: (1987): ". . . a collectivity of people with a high degree of formality of structure working together to meet a goal or goals." (p. 477). Covers many topics.	Author quotes Daft (1998): "Organizations are '(1) social entities that (2) are goal directed, (3) are designed as deliberately structured and coordinated activity systems, and (4) are linked to the external environment.'" (p. 87) Covers most topics. Focus on soc. serv. orgs.	"Large group theory and research, however, are generally limited to the study of organizations or, more properly, bureaucracy. The terms bureaucracy refers to any relatively complex and formal organization." (p. 332) Covers few topics.

	Hutchison, E. (2003b)	Kirst-Ashman, K. (2000)	Longres, J. (2000)
Community– Definition and # of topics covered.	". . . community is people bound either by geography or by webs of communication, sharing common ties, and interacting with one another." (p. 513) Covers many topics.	Author quotes Homan (1994): "A community is a number of people who have something in common with one another that connects them in some way and that distinguishes them from others.'" (p. 29) Covers most topics.	"A community is a type of social system that is distinguished by the personal or affective nature of the ties that hold its members together. It is groups of people who sense a common identity, bond with one another, and become attached to or affiliated with one another through regular interaction." (p. 75) Covers many topics.
Number of syllabi citing text	7	7	27
Impressions	Excellent balance of HB & SE and theory & practice.	Comprehensive, clear, and concise.	Excellent integration of complicated concepts without being overwhelming.

General Description of Systems HB&SE Textbooks

	Pillari, V. & Newsome, M. (1998)	Schriver, J. (2001)
Text Structure	This 228 page text is one of two companion texts. The other text focuses on individual life span. This text focuses on systems & is divided into 5 chapters: *Overview of systems *Families *Groups *Organizations *Communities Each chapter ends with a section on implications for social work practice and further reading/video suggestions	The 576 page text is divided into ten chapters: *Intro *Traditional and alternative paradigms *Paradigm thinking *Traditional perspectives: individuals *Alternative perspectives: individuals *Familiness *Groups *Organizations *Communities *Conclusion Each chapter emphasizes "traditional and alternative perspective"" on each topic. Each chapter also includes an "Internet Search Guide" that gives the reader a suggested list of search terms for finding more information about the concepts presented in the chapter & "illustrative reading"–a scholarly essay or excerpt of a book that provides a specific example of the material discussed in the chapter.
Audience	BSW, MSW	BSW, MSW
Theory Explication	Emphasizes ecological perspective.	Theoretical explanations and debates are highlighted throughout the text. Chapters 1-3 focus on theoretical background knowledge and debate. Early in Chapter 1 (p. 6), Schriver defines traditional and alternative paradigms. He then goes on to discuss critical thinking and deconstruction in the subsequent pages. The second chapter presents the positivism as the dominant epistemological paradigm and intuitive, interpretive, and subjective ways of knowing as the alternative paradigms.
Major Themes	*diversity *oppression *patriarchy *feminism	*social justice *poverty *critical thinking

	Pillari, V. & Newsome, M. (1998)	Schriver, J. (2001)
Theory for Practice	Though each chapter includes an "Implications for practice" section, this section does not emphasize skill development.	There is a 2-page section on assessment and a text box teaching skills for strengths-based practice, but skills are not emphasized systematically.
Definition of the Social Environment	Not clearly stated.	Rather than giving a specific definition of SE, the author gives examples: "If the social environment is primary and human behavior is secondary... We might begin by trying to understand the important influences of the larger social environment - the community, for example, or society or culture..." (p. 10) The book addresses the SE vs. HB debate directly in the introduction and in the first chapter on individuals. Throughout the rest of the book, the acronym SEHB is often substituted for HBSE.
Structures of the Social Environment	*Families *Organizations *Groups *Communities	*Families *Organizations *Groups *Communities

SE in Systems HB&SE Textbooks

	Pillari, V. & Newsome, M. (1998)	Schriver, J. (2001)
Social Problems & Societal Focus	The first chapter includes sections on diversity, feminism, oppression, and patriarchy. The chapter on families includes a section about families living in poverty. Each chapter includes human diversity content.	In the first chapter, Schriver discusses poverty reduction, oppression, and global poverty as priorities for social work in the present and future. The focus on social problems is echoed throughout the text. Human diversity issues are discussed in every chapter of the book.
Social Justice & Social Work Values	Though the text implies certain social work values through its emphasis on diversity & oppression, it does not directly address social work values by referring to the code of ethics in the introduction or by including a separate section on social work values.	In the first chapter, Schriver quotes the NASW Code of Ethics, citing the sections on social justice and related values as cornerstones of the profession. The focus on values is echoed throughout the text.
Family– Definition and # of topics covered.	The authors cite Meyer (1990): "Two or more people who are joined together by bonds of intimacy." (p. 34) Covers most topics.	"Familiness includes the traditional functions and responsibilities assigned by societies to families, such as childbearing, childrearing, intimacy, and security. It also recognizes the great diversity in structures, values, and contexts that define family for different people." (p. 317) Covers many topics.
Groups– Definition and # of topics covered.	"A group consists of two or more people interacting in such a manner that each is influenced by every other." (p. 89) Covers many topics.	Citing Brown (1991) and Johnson & Johnson (1991), Schriver defines groups as being characterized by "shared purpose and common interaction" (p. 392). Covers many topics.

	Pillari, V. & Newsome, M. (1998)	Schriver, J. (2001)
Organizations–Definition and # of topics covered.	Focus on SW orgs. The authors cite definitions by Kamerman (1983), Austin & Hasenfeld (1985), and Bellah, Madsen, Sullivan, Swidler, & Tipton (1985): "Social welfare organizations are formal organizations legitimized by the state to deliver personal social services and other benefits and goods to citizens, participate in deviance control on behalf of the state, and promote the public interest or common welfare." (p. 131) Covers many topics.	Schriver uses a number of perspectives to define organizations (Etzioni (1964), Parsons, Gortner, Mahler, & Nicholson (1987), and comments that the common theme in these perspectives is that they "recognize organizations as collectives of people working together to accomplish a goal (or goals)." (p. 435). Covers many topics.
Community–Definition and # of topics covered.	". . . a number of people with common ties and interests." (p. 174). Covers few topics.	Schriver writes that there are multiple definitions of community, but settles on "a collective of people. This *includes individuals, groups, organizations, and families; shared interests; regular interaction to fulfill shared interests through informal and formally organized means; and some degree of mutual identification among members as belonging to the collective.*" (Emphasis in original. p. 502) Covers most topics.
Number of syllabi citing text	6	31
Impressions	Seems appropriate for readers with a limited social science background.	Very comprehensive with good balance between HB and SE.

APPENDIX 3. General Description of Theory HB&SE Textbooks

	Bloom, M. & Klein, W. (1997)	Greene, R. (1999)	Robbins, S., Chatterjee, P., & Canda, E. (1998)
Text Structure	The 297 page text is divided into three sections: *Theory–which theories to include and how to include them in HBSE courses *Content–what HBSE courses should cover *Teaching–how to teach an effective HBSE course; what HBSE teaches students This text has a unique structure. The individual chapters pose core questions about the teaching of HBSE at the graduate level, and scholars on opposing sides of the debate answer each question. Each chapter begins with a very brief (1-2 paragraphs) synopsis of the debate and then an introduction to the scholars featured (scholarly interests, professional associations, etc.)	This 436 page text is divided into 11 chapters: *HB Theory, Person-in-Environment, and SW Method *HB Theory and SW Practice *Freudian Theory *Eriksonian Theory *Carl Rogers and the Person-Centered Approach *Cognitive Theory for SW Practice *General Systems Theory *Ecological Perspective *Social Construction *Feminist Theory *Genetics, Environment, and Development Each chapter (except for chapters 1 and 2, which are treated as one) is followed by a critique of the theory presented in that chapter. Each chapter follows a similar structure; includes an introduction to the theory, cross-cultural considerations, and implications for social work practice.	This 465 page text is divided into 13 chapters: *The Nature of Theories *Systems Theory *Conflict Theories *Theories of Empowerment *Theories of Assimilation, Acculturation, and Bicultural Socialization *Psychodynamic Theory *Theories of Life Span Development *Theories of Cognitive and Moral Development *Symbolic Interaction *Phenomenology, Social Constructionism, and Hermeneutics *Behaviorism, Social Learning, and Exchange Theory *Transpersonal Theory *Application of Theories Each chapter, except the first and last, follows a similar structure: Historical context, key concepts, contemporary issues, application to social work practice, critical analysis, consistency with social work values and ethics, philosophical underpinnings, methodological issues and empirical support, and summary.

	Bloom, M. & Klein, W. (1997)	Greene, R. (1999)	Robbins, S., Chatterjee, P., & Canda, E. (1998)
Audience	Not specifically identified.	Not specifically identified.	BSW, MSW
Theory Explication	The text begins with a discussion of whether post-positivism is an appropriate epistemological framework for HBSE courses. The remainder of Part I of the book includes other theoretical discussions, including teaching the strengths perspective, stage theories, and the teaching of critical thinking.	The first chapter deals primarily with epistemological issues and introduces positivist, post-positivist, and postmodern approaches. It also addresses the importance of human behavior theory to social work practice (as an organizing tool for assessment & intervention, as a means to professional practice, & as an organizing framework.)	Chapter 1 gives students several tools for beginning to think about theory, including a discussion of what theory is, types of theory (micro, mezzo, macro), the construction of theory in an ideological context, and the application of theory to practice.
Major Themes	Because of the structure of the text, the overarching theme is that multiple perspectives are required in understanding HBSE issues.	Examines the universality of a given theory, its ability to explain phenomena for diverse communities, and its definition of pathology and health. Critical thinking emphasized.	The overarching theme of this text is to teach students how to critically evaluate theory in a social work context.
Theory for Practice	Not directly addressed.	Each chapter includes a "Direct Practice in Social Work" section, but these sections seem to summarize the material in a social work context rather than discussing specific skills for implementation.	The application to social work sections of the chapter teach some skills based on the theories presented in the chapter using a flowchart. The flowcharts help students define & assess SW situations.
Definition of the Social Environment	Not clearly stated.	Not clearly stated.	Not clearly stated.
Structures of the Social Environment	Not clearly stated.	Not clearly stated.	*individuals *groups *families *organizations *institutions *communities

SE in Theory HB&SE Textbooks

	Bloom, M. & Klein, W. (1997)	Greene, R. (1999)	Robbins, S., Chatterjee, P., & Canda, E. (1998)
Social Problems & Societal Focus	The text includes chapters on diversity and feminist content, whether to include international issues in HBSE, and whether to include religion and spirituality issues in HBSE.	Not directly addressed.	Chapters 4 and 5 discuss oppression, feminist theory, lesbian, and gay empowerment theories, immigration, and biculturalism.

APPENDIX 3 (continued)

	Bloom, M. & Klein, W. (1997)	Greene, R. (1999)	Robbins, S., Chatterjee, P., & Canda, E. (1998)
Social Justice & Social Work Values	Not directly addressed.	In Chapter 2, Greene quotes the CWSE curriculum policy in social work education diversity for MSW students, which comments on the need to address social and economic justice and populations-at-risk. She also quotes the NASW code of ethics, including sections on ethical principles, the value of promoting social justice, and cultural competence.	Each chapter includes a section on the theory's consistency with social work values and ethics. These 1-2 page sections describe how well the theory corresponds to specific social work values.
Family– Definition and # of topics covered.	Not clearly stated. Covers few topics.	In a separate text box, Greene offers 6 definitions of family, to show how concepts of family have changed over time, from Billingsley's (1968) focus on families consisting of married partners and children to The White House Conference on Aging's (1981) definition: 'A family is a system of related and unrelated individuals integrated by patterns of social relationships and mutual help.' (p. 50) Covers few topics.	Not clearly stated. Covers few topics.
Groups– Definition and # of topics covered.	Not clearly stated. Covers few topics.	Not clearly stated. Covers few topics.	Not clearly stated. Covers few topics.
Organizations– Definition and # of topics covered.	Not clearly stated. Covers few topics.	Not clearly stated. Covers few topics.	Not clearly stated. Covers few topics.
Community– Definition and # of topics covered.	Not clearly stated. Covers few topics.	Not clearly stated. Covers few topics.	Not clearly stated. Covers few topics.
Number of syllabi citing text	2	17	25
Impressions	Useful for advanced HBSE courses.	Useful for advanced HBSE courses.	Excellent balance between theory and practice.

Reflecting on the Social Environment Dimensions of HB&SE: An HB&SE Faculty Member as Discussant

Susan Stone

SUMMARY. This paper discusses the contributions of three studies of the Human Behavior and the Social Environment curriculum presented in this volume (Mulroy & Austin; Taylor, Mulroy, & Austin; Taylor, Austin, & Mulroy). A key theme across these theoretical and empirical pieces is that content related to social environment may not be coherently or consistently presented across courses. This finding is discussed in light of the general move toward contextualism in the social sciences in recent decades. Implications for social work pedagogy, research, and theory development are discussed. *[Article copies available for a fee from The Haworth Document Delivery Service: 1-800-HAWORTH. E-mail address: <docdelivery@haworthpress.com> Website: <http://www.HaworthPress.com> © 2004 by The Haworth Press, Inc. All rights reserved.]*

KEYWORDS. Human behavior and the social environment, social work education, contextualism

---

Susan Stone, PhD, is Assistant Professor, School of Social Welfare, University of California, Berkeley.

[Haworth co-indexing entry note]: "Reflecting on the Social Environment Dimensions of HB&SE: An HB&SE Faculty Member as Discussant." Stone, Susan. Co-published simultaneously in *Journal of Human Behavior in the Social Environment* (The Haworth Social Work Practice Press, an imprint of The Haworth Press, Inc.) Vol. 10, No. 3, 2004, pp. 111-118; and: *The Conundrum of Human Behavior in the Social Environment* (ed: Marvin D. Feit and John S. Wodarski) The Haworth Social Work Practice Press, an imprint of The Haworth Press, Inc., 2004, pp. 111-118. Single or multiple copies of this article are available for a fee from The Haworth Document Delivery Service [1-800-HAWORTH, 9:00 a.m. - 5:00 p.m. (EST). E-mail address: docdelivery@haworthpress.com].

© 2004 by The Haworth Press, Inc. All rights reserved.
Digital Object Identifier: 10.1300/J137v10n03_05

There are two salient points of contention related to the Human Behavior and Social Environment (HBSE) curriculum: (1) the bodies of knowledge that constitute its philosophical, theoretical and empirical foundations, and (2) the scope of content that is covered (Klein & Bloom, 1997). It should neither be particularly alarming nor surprising that contention exists when it comes to conceptualizing the complex nature and consequences of interactions between human behaviors and their social environments. Wakefield's critique of the ecological perspective (Wakefield 1996a; 1996b), for example, captures the central theoretical challenges inherent in this endeavor.

Given the inherent complexity associated with this area of the curriculum, it is quite surprising that there is a paucity of primary research that actually addresses or helps to inform these issues. It is also surprising that there is so little dialogue in the field about such a central area of the social work curriculum. The last formalized debate on these issues occurred nearly ten years ago (Klein & Bloom, 1997). Clearly, the extent to which there is consensus within these has tremendous implications for curriculum development and pedagogy. The absence of dialogue also raises questions about progress in theoretical development in the larger social work/social welfare field.

These three papers by Michael Austin, Elizabeth Mulroy, and Sarah Taylor have the potential to reinvigorate both debate and research in this area. In total, the papers address two aspects of the curriculum, namely its conceptual underpinnings related to the social environment (Mulroy & Austin, 2004) and the variability in course and textbooks (Taylor, Austin, & Mulroy, 2004; Taylor, Mulroy, & Austin, 2004). Because the topics addressed by these papers fit neatly into areas of contention identified by Klein and Bloom (1997), I will discuss them within their framework (bodies of knowledge and scope of content) in order to raise questions and implications for curriculum development and the field as a whole.

NATURE AND CHARACTER OF THE KNOWLEDGE BASE

Mulroy and Austin (2004) argue that renewed attention should be placed on the social environment because the very nature of social environments or communities has fundamentally changed. Using Roland Warren's (1963) definition of microsystems (local communities) and macrosystems (larger socio-structural forces), they highlight how globalization and rapid demographic and technological change have fundamentally reshaped local communities and, by implication, the nature and quality of interactions between persons and environments. They present a framework that outlines key dimensions relevant to the structure of and inter-relationships between the macro-system and micro-system. In short, the framework addresses how larger social forces relate to the local communities in which individuals are embedded.

The contributions of this framework are several. First, it is comprehensive. Second, it is theoretically neutral. One could potentially locate any domain-specific, socio-structural theory or concept within it (i.e., determine what aspects of or interrelationships between the macro and micro system it addresses). In this respect, it is an analytic tool with which one could critically assess the utility of a particular theory or set of theories in understanding the nature and quality of the macro- and micro-systemic interrelationships. The HBSE curriculum typically presents ecological or eco-systemic perspectives that describes that individuals are nested in multi-layered environments. This framework paints a detailed portrait of horizontal and vertical linkages between communities, and larger, often unobservable social forces (e.g., globalization).

It is also important to consider the contribution of this framework to addressing the inconsistency of how the social environment is conceptualized and operationalized across actual courses and texts (Taylor, Austin & Mulroy, 2004; Taylor, Mulroy, & Austin, 2004). This framework provides a way to operationalize the term "environment."

It is also important to note two items that Austin, Mulroy, and Taylor do not address. First, there has not only been real change in social environments over recent decades, but there has also been a great deal of change in how social scientists conceptualize and think about social environments. Most of the social sciences–and especially related to the human services–have become more "contextualist" over the last few decades. That is to say, they have moved beyond the question of whether environments matter to the question of how and why they do.

Second, Austin, Mulroy, and Taylor rightly point out (and present evidence to this effect) that the relative emphasis of the HBSE curriculum is focused on human behavior in settings nested *within* a given community (e.g., individuals, families, small groups) rather than interrelationships between them and larger macro-systemic forces. However, CSWE standards suggest that the HBSE curriculum address the "ways social systems promote or deter people in maintaining health or well-being." While the authors help us define what is actually meant by the term "social systems," they acknowledge that they are not explicitly addressing links between these macro and micro systemic processes of the social environment and individual processes of human behavior. I would argue that this is an extremely critical link, referred in the CSWE standards as the reciprocal interaction between human behavior and the social environment.

Both these points, in my opinion, relate to the character of the empirical base. Related to the first point, some would argue that while social scientists pay a good deal of "lip service" to the importance of environments, available research does not often reflect this conceptual emphasis. In other words, it is very difficult to locate research that is actually matched to the thick conceptual description outlined by Mulroy and Austin (2004). More specifically, we rarely ask questions that attempt to link larger historical or economic forces to individual behavior and functioning. It is not because these are not key questions, but because they are very difficult to research. An important exception is the life course research of Elder who seeks to document how individual lives were altered in periods of economic downturns, such as the Great Depression and, more recently, during farming crises in Iowa (Elder & Caspi 1991; Conger et al., 2001). An important finding of this research is that macro-systems forces exert an influence on individual behavior through changes in family social support structures. It is important to note that an even smaller body of research addresses "reciprocal" interactions between persons and environments. Mulroy and Austin (2004) focus primarily on uni-directional or downward processes linking larger societal forces to microsystem patterns. It is also clear that there may be upward processes, as well. Michael Lewis (2002) argues forcibly that the social sciences do not yet possess empirical methods to adequately answer reciprocity-related questions.

Scope and Emphasis

While the authors point out the limitations of using course syllabi as a measure of HBSE course coverage, the heterogeneity among course outlines is quite staggering. Their findings also are consistent with other recent analyses of the HBSE curriculum (Farley et al., 2002). Their set of papers raise the question of *why* there is so much variation and whether it matters. At best, heterogeneity means that there is an overall lack of consensus as to how to approach the conceptual underpinnings of the course (see Farley et al., 2002). At worst, it means that social work students may not exposed to a common set of foundational knowledge across programs or courses within programs. It is notable that certain types of course outlines are more tightly coupled with CSWE standards than others.

It is perhaps more interesting to ask why there is so much variation. Because Taylor, Austin, and Mulroy (2004) obtained a fairly "mixed" sample of social work programs (in terms of region, size, type), their findings can not be easily explained by different school characteristics. They do, however, find that programs allocate different amounts of time to the HBSE curriculum. This might suggest that the amount of time to cover material is an important source of variation. This variation could reflect disagreement about the intersection of human behavior and the social environment (e.g., direct/practice versus indirect/policy perspectives). Or, this variation could simply reflect the inherent complexity of the subject matter. Having a good understanding of the actual source of variation is a critical piece of a future HB&SE research agenda.

They also find that they could classify HBSE courses and textbooks according to one of three clusters: lifespan, systems, or theory oriented. In their discussions, they largely present these findings as reflecting program-level idiosyncracies related to the selection of topics (e.g., discipline-related preferences of particular programs or instructors). I would argue that these findings might speak to a larger substantive problem. That is, differences in clusters may reflect that there are three interrelated, yet independent components of the HBSE curriculum: an understanding of the general pathways of persons lives over time, an outline of general systems components, and a critical theory component. They cite evidence, in fact, that suggests that over time the course has evolved to progressively incorporate more and more content that is thought to be central to the curriculum. This is an issue that cuts across programs and suggests that social work–as a discipline–needs to reconsider what constitutes key foundation HB&SE knowledge for social work practice at both the direct and indirect levels of practice.

IMPLICATIONS

These authors are quite clear about some of the limitations of the empirical findings they generated. It goes without saying that more research is sorely needed in this area. In particular, studies which replicate these findings with the population of MSW programs and using multiple methods (e.g., class observations) to look at actual content coverage would be especially useful first steps. The relative emphasis on the social environment and the variability across courses suggest an important set of implications related to the HBSE curriculum, the role of the Council on Social Work Education, and the state of the field.

Implications related to the curriculum: I would argue that there are two key issues raised that are specific to HBSE curriculum development. First, Mulroy, and Austin (2004) underscore the importance and utility of carefully specifying the elements of mapping out the structure and processes of both human behavior and social environment. These maps remind us about the nature and scope of the terrain that needs to be covered in order to fully grapple with so-called "reciprocal" relationships between individuals and their environments. In essence, do we focus attention on describing versus explaining what is meant by human behavior and the social environment and what are the trade-offs associated with either perspective? An argument for description over explanation is that the nature and quality of interactions between individuals and environments are constantly in flux over time and will likely require flexible explanatory systems. Careful mapping or describing may better enable us to: (1) maintain a spirit of pluralism with respect to potential theoretical models, and (2) critically assess the utility of specific models.

A second and related issue is whether there should be a shift in attention to the state of theoretical and empirical development in the field at large. In other words, should there be a move to "theory-oriented" HBSE courses that critically evaluate the extent to which the current knowledge base actually aids us in navigating this complex map. Stated another way, the role of the HBSE curriculum would assess the degree to which the literature enables us to answer macro and micro questions about individual behavior (e.g., by what mechanisms do forces related to globalization influence communities and how do community changes, in turn, impact individual functioning). This type of curricular emphasis could provide clearer relationships for how students are taught how to use "theory for practice." It is also more tightly coupled with the current emphasis in the social work profession on evidence- or empirically-based practice and policies.

Council on Social Work Education Standards and Criteria: A critical assessment of the CSWE curriculum statement on HBSE content (Taylor, Austin, & Mulroy, 2004) reveals a fundamental failure to grapple with the state of the social science empirical base. As I noted above, there is virtually no literature that informs "the reciprocal relationships between human behavior and social environments." However, there is literature that looks at unidirectional relationships between persons and environments. The school effects literature (Bryk & Raudenbush, 1992) and the neighborhood effects literature (Sampson et al., 2002) are exemplars. These are not bodies of evidence that are typically referred to in HBSE texts. Overall, these literatures suggest that while characteristics of particular social systems do have relationships to individual health and well-being, the overall magnitude of effects are quite small. To go back to Elder's work, the effects of larger social systems seem to impact individuals indirectly through the influences of the proximate, small group settings (e.g., families and relationships).

It is clearly problematic that rich, broad conceptualizations of the social environment remain at the margin of the HBSE curriculum. This reality does not reflect current shift in the social sciences to document the contexts for understanding human behavior. It also raises the question of whether CSWE is putting in place appropriate criteria and enabling guidelines to reflect the reciprocal nature of human behavior and the social environment which constitute such a central part of the social work mission.

Implications for the field: As social work educators, we should not be particularly alarmed that there would be debates about the conceptual and empirical foundations of the field. Our profession attempts to impact the well-being of individuals by taking into account the attributes of individuals and their environments. These attributes are not static; they are in flux in real and historical time and space. These issues pose substantial theoretical and research challenges (see Sameroff, 2003 for a discussion of these). It is clear that the HBSE curriculum does not challenge students in this respect. What is potentially more disheartening is that we are not explicitly engaging in these challenges as a field. The current state of the HBSE curriculum, the lack of research informing it, and the absence of dialogue may be symptomatic of increasingly balkanized curriculum with little attention to the scholarship of teaching and curriculum development that seems to pervade the field and our own faculties.

REFERENCES

Conger, R.D., & Conger, K.J. (2002). Resilience in midwestern families. Selected findings from the first decade of a prospective, longitudinal study. *Journal of Marriage & the Family, 64*(2), 361-73.
Elder, G. H., & Caspi, A. (1988). Economic stress in lives: Developmental perspectives. *Journal of Social Issues, 44*(4), 25-45.
Farley, O., Smith, L. Boyle, S., & Ronnau, J. (2002). A review of foundation MSW human behavior courses. *Journal of Human Behavior in the Social Environment, 6*(2), 1-12.

Klein, W., & Bloom, M. (1997). *Controversial issues in human behavior in the social environment*. Boston: Allyn & Bacon.

Lewis, M. (2000). Toward a development of psychopathology: Models, definitions, and prediction. In Sameroff, A.J., Lewis, M., & Miller, S.M. (Eds.), *Handbook of developmental psychopathology* (2nd ed.), (pp. 3-22). New York: Kluwer Academic Press.

Mulroy, E., & Austin, M.J. (2004). Towards a comprehensive framework for understanding the social environment: In search of theory for practice. *Journal of Human Behavior in the Social Environment*, *10*(3), 25-59.

Raudenbush, S. W., & Bryk, A. S. (2002). *Hierarchical linear models: Applications and data analysis methods*. Thousand Oaks, CA: Sage Publications.

Sameroff, A.J. (2000). Dialectical processes in developmental psychopathology. In Sameroff, A.J., Lewis, M., & Miller, S.M. (Eds.), *Handbook of developmental psychopathology* (2nd ed.), (pp. 23-40). New York: Kluwer Academic Press.

Sampson, R. J., Morenoff, J. D., & Gannon-Rowley, T. (2002). Assessing "neighborhood effects": Social processes and new directions in research. *Annual Review of Sociology*, *28*, 443-478.

Taylor, S., Austin, M.J., & Mulroy, E. (2004). Evaluating the social environment component of social work courses on human behavior and the social environment. *Journal of Human Behavior in the Social Environment*, *10*(3), 61-84.

Taylor, S., Mulroy, E., & Austin, M.J. (2004). Social work textbooks on human behavior and the social environment: An analysis of the social environment component. *Journal of Human Behavior in the Social Environment*, *10*(3), 85-109.

Wakefield, J. (1996a). Does social work need the eco-systems perspective? Part 1. Is the perspective clinically useful? *Social Service Review*, *70*(1), 1-32.

Wakefield, J. (1996b). Does social work need the eco-systems perspective? Part 2. Does the perspective save social work from incoherence? *Social Service Review*, *70*(2), 183-213.

Warren, R. (1963). *The community in America*. Chicago: Rand McNally.

Index

Numbers followed by "f" indicate figures; "t" following a page number indicates tabular material.

"Aging, Slow-Growing Heartland" states, 36
American Association of Schools of Social Work, 3
Austin, M.J., 25,61,72,73,73f,74f,76,83-84, 85,89,92,92f,93f,94,112-116

Bloom, M., 112
Bowman, V.E., 9
Brooks, W., 64,65-66,71,72

Change, in social environment, 50-51
Charity Organizations, 2
Coalition politics, in macro-system perspective of social environment, 40
Combination HBSE course outline, 79
Community groups, in micro-system perspective of social environment, 45-46,46f
Community neighborhoods, in micro-system perspective of social environment, 44
Community-based organizations, in micro-system perspective of social environment, 44-45
Conflict, in social environment, 50-51
Cosmopolitan(s), 50
Council on Social Work Education (CSWE), 2,3,26,61,63,65,74-76,85

defined, 3
Education Policy and Accreditation Standards of, 3
standards and criteria of, 116-117
Council on Social Work Education (CSWE) HBSE standards, 70-71
Craig, G., 31
CSWE. *See* Council on Social Work Education (CSWE)

Delucia, J.L., 9
Demone, H., Jr., 37
Development, stages of, described, 47
Diversity, 48-49
Downs, A., 29,32
Dulmus, C.N., 6
Dwyer, D., 6
Dziegieleski, S.F., 4,10

Economy, political, 35-37
Elder, G.H., 114
Environment(s), social, comprehensive framework for understanding, 25-59. *See also* Social environment, comprehensive framework for understanding
Evidence-based practices, websites targeting, 23-24

Fabricant, M., 37

Farley, O., 65-66,71,72,74
Fields, D., 55
Fisher, R., 37
Frey, W., 36

Gibbs, P., 87
Gibelman, M., 37
Gil, D., 30
Global interdependencies, 36
Gottdiener, M., 35-36
Gray, B., 28,38,40
Great Depression, 114

HAC. *See* Housing Assistance
    Corporation (HAC)
Harvey, D., 31
Hasenfeld, Y., 50
HBSE. *See* Human behavior and social
    environment (HBSE)
Healey, L., 36
Homelessness, HAC response to,
    41,42f-43f
Housing Assistance Corporation
    (HAC), 28,41,42f-43f,54-56
  response to homelessness,
    41,42f-43f
Human behavior, social work courses
    on, evaluating social
    environment in, 61-84
Human behavior and social
    environment (HBSE),
    1-25,61-63,74-77
  criteria in, application of, 70
  curriculum for, 1-25
    evidence-based, literature review
      for, 4-10
  discussion of, 71-72
  implications for, 10-12
  prototype course outlines, 71
  social environment components of,
    72-73,73f,74f
  social environment dimensions of
    emphasis of, 114-115
    implications of, 115-117
    knowledge base in, nature and
      character of, 112-115
    reflections on, 111-118
    scope of, 114-115
  social work courses on, social
    environment in, 61-84. *See
    also* Social environment, in
    social work courses on HBSE
  social work textbooks on, 85-110
    findings in, 90-91
    introduction to, 86-87
    life cycle of, described, 98-103
    method of analysis in, 89-90
    systems-based, described,
      103-108
    theory-based, described,
      108-110
  syllabi for, 21-23
Human behavior and social
    environment (HBSE)
    course(s), types of, 68-70,69t
Human behavior and social
    environment (HBSE) course
    outline, 79
  lifespan-oriented, 80
  systems-oriented, 82
  theory-oriented, 81
*Human Behavior in the Social
    Environment–Integrating
    Theory and Evidence-Based
    Practice,* 4
Human growth and development
  biology and genetics in, 4-5
  cognitive theory, 6
  group level variables, 9
  group perspective to, 7-10
  individual perspective to, 4-7
  labeling theory, 7
  learning theories, 7-8
  life span perspective, 6-7
  macro-level variables, 9-10
  social exchange, 8-9
Hunter, M., 63

Hunt-Jackson, J., 6

Institutional failures, 33
Integrating mechanisms, in social environment, 51-52
Inter-organizational service networks, in macro-system perspective of social environment, 39

Johnson, M.M., 12

Kanter, R.M., 39
Klein, W., 112

Lauber, H., 53
Lawrence, S.A., 5
Leadership, in social environment, 49-50
Leo, C.M., 9
Levande, D., 62,64
Lewis, M., 114
Lifespan-oriented HBSE course outline, 80
Local(s), 50
Longres, J., 30

Maccio, E.M., 9
Macro-system, 26-27
Mailick, M., 63,64
"Melting Pot" states, 36
Micro-system, 26-27
Milford Conference, 2
Moote, G., Jr., 8
Mulroy, E.A., 25,53,61,72,73,73f,74f,76,83-84,85,89,92,92f,93f,94,112-116

National Association of Schools of Social Administration, 3
"New Sunbelt" states, 36

Organization(s), groups in, in micro-system perspective of social environment, 45-46,46f

People changing organizations, 45
People processing organizations, 44-45
People sustaining organizations, 45
Personal Responsibility and Work Opportunity Reconciliation Act of 1996, 34
Pickvance, C., 35-36
Politic(s), coalition, in macro-system perspective of social environment, 40
Political economy, 35-37
Power, in social environment, 49-50
Practitioner-environment interaction, in social environment, 52-53
Privatization, 36-37
Process
    defined, 43
    elements of, 49-53
Public/private/partnerships, in macro-system perspective of social environment, 38-39

Rapp-Pagilicci, L., 8-9
Rawls, J., 30,31
Reyes, L.A., 12
Rhodes, R., 12

Saleebey, D., 63
Scanlon, E., 30
Schorr, A., 34-35,37
Smith, K.D., 9

Social environment
  change in, 50-51
  comprehensive framework for understanding, 25-59
    political economy, 35-37
    social policies, 33-35
    social problems, 31-33
  conflict in, 50-51
  implications for, 53-56
  integrating mechanisms in, 51-52
  leadership in, 49-50
  macro-system perspective of, 27-28,28f,29-41
    coalition politics, 40
    collective responses as mediating structures, 37-41
    inter-organizational service networks, 39
    public/private/partnerships, 38-39
    social justice, 30-31
    societal forces in, 30-37
  micro-system(s) of, described, 43
  micro-system perspective of, 41-46,42f-43f,46f
    community-based organizations, 44-45
    community groups, 45-46,46f
    community neighborhoods, 44
    organizational groups, 45-46,46f
    process of, 43-46,46f
    structure of, 43-46,46f
  power in, 49-50
  practitioner-environment interaction in, 52-53
  process of, elements of, 49-53
  in social work courses on HBSE, 61-84
    findings of, 67-73,68f,69t,73f,74f
    implications of, 74-77
    literature review, 63-66
    methods of, 66-67
  structure of, elements of, 47-49

Social environment dimensions, of HBSE, reflections on, 111-118
Social environment framework, case vignette, 53-55
Social justice, 30-31
  territorial, 31
Social policies, 33-35
Social problems, 31-33
Social work textbooks, on HBSE, 85-110. *See also* Human behavior and social environment (HBSE), social work textbooks on
Societal forces, in macro-system perspective of social environment, 30-37. *See also specific type*
  political economy, 35-37
  social justice, 30-31
  social policies, 33-35
  social problems, 31-33
Solomon, R., 30
Spero, 87
Stages of development, described, 47
Stamm, 87
Stone, S., 111
Structure
  defined, 43
  diversity in, 48-49
  elements of, 47-49
  stages of development in, 47
  systems of exchange in, 47-48
Success, normative definitions of, 55-56
Sullivan, M., 7
Sutton, 87
Systems of exchange, 47-48
Systems-oriented HBSE course outline, 82

Taylor, S., 61,85,89,112,113,115
Territorial social justice, 31

Theory-oriented HBSE course outline, 81

United Nations Development Program, 32
Urban Problems and Prospects, 29
Urban restructuring, 35-36
U.S. Census for 2000, 36

Vance, 63
Vigilante, F., 63,64

Warren, R., 26,35,112
Weil, M., 48
Wodarski, J.S., 1,4,10
Wolch, J., 37

Yalom, I.D., 9

Zittel-Palamara, K., 5